student resource manual to accompany

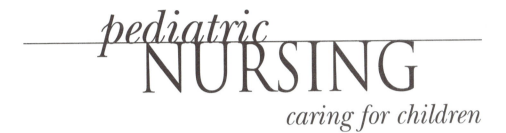

pediatric NURSING
caring for children

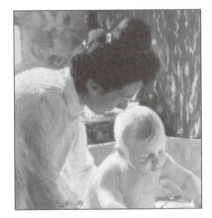

second edition

Cathleen M. Homrighaus, RN, MSN
Faculty, Pediatric Nursing
St. Joseph's Hospital Health Center
School of Nursing
Syracuse, New York

D0022396

Appleton & Lange
Stamford, Connecticut

Copyright © 1999 by Appleton & Lange

www.appletonlange.com

99 00 01 02 03/ 10 9 8 7 6 5 4 3 2 1

Prentice Hall International (UK) Limited, *London*
Prentice Hall of Australia Pty. Limited, *Sydney*
Prentice Hall Canada, Inc., *Toronto*
Prentice Hall Hispanoamericana, S.A., *Mexico*
Prentice Hall of India Private Limited, *New Delhi*
Prentice Hall of Japan, Inc., *Tokyo*
Simon & Schuster Asia Pte. Ltd., *Singapore*
Editora Prentice Hall do Brasil Ltda., *Rio de Janeiro*
Prentice Hall, *Upper Saddle River, New Jersey*

ISBN: 0-8385-8168-4

Acquisitions Editor: David P. Carroll
Designer: Libby Schmitz

PRINTED IN THE UNITED STATES OF AMERICA

CONTENTS

Nurse's Role in Care of the Ill and Injured Child: Hospital, Community Settings, and Home

Chapter Overview

Chapter 1 presents a general introduction to the care of children in a family-oriented context. Topics discussed include the role of the nurse in pediatrics, the nursing process, and settings for pediatric nursing care. A discussion of the contemporary climate for pediatric care focuses on cultural considerations, morbidity and mortality statistics, and current health care issues. Legal concepts and responsibilities of nurses regarding nursing practice regulation, accountability, and risk management are introduced. Finally, legal and ethical issues in the practice of pediatric nursing are presented.

Learning Objectives

After studying this chapter, you should be able to:
- Discuss the role of the nurse in pediatric practice.
- List five possible settings for pediatric nursing practice.
- Identify the key elements of family-centered care.
- Describe the impact of a family's culture on the care of a child.
- Interpret the mortality and morbidity statistics for children.
- Discuss how mortality and morbidity statistics can be used in pediatric nursing practice.

- Discuss the impact of research, lifesaving technology, and health care financing on the family and society.
- Outline the benefits of home care for chronically ill children.
- Explain how pediatric nurses assume responsibiilty and accountability for their practice.
- Summarize the nursing information that must be documented in a patient's record.
- Describe the nurse's role in obtaining informed consent.
- Discuss the ethical decision-making process.

Review of Concepts

Matching

Match the items in list 1 with the appropriate definition or phrase in list 2. (*Note:* Terms may be used more than once.)

1. Role of Nurse in Pediatric Care

List 1
A. Direct nursing care
B. Patient education
C. Patient advocacy
D. Case management

LIST 2
1. _____ Informing parents about home care services
2. _____ Giving medications
3. _____ Discharge planning
4. _____ Preparing child and parents for procedures
5. _____ Ensuring that child's rights are upheld in the hospital
6. _____ Providing family support
7. _____ Referring family to financial counselors
8. _____ Providing anticipatory guidance about child's future development
9. _____ Referring family to a home care agency

2. Regulation of Nursing Practice

LIST 1
A. "Baby Doe" regulations
B. National Organ Transplant Act
C. Advance directives
D. Risk management
E. Quality assurance
F. Nurse Practice Act
G. Standards of Nursing Practice
H. Infant mortality
I. Morbidity

LIST 2
1. _____ Living will
2. _____ Illness or injury that results in a chronic condition
3. _____ Monitors outcomes of care to measure compliance with standards of care
4. _____ Regulates instances when death of one child may benefit another child
5. _____ Death occurring during first year of life
6. _____ Protects rights of infants with severe defects
7. _____ Compliance with standards to decrease liability
8. _____ Defines legal roles and responsibilities of nurses
9. _____ Public and patient responsibilities for which nurses are accountable

SHORT ESSAY

1. Family-centered care is an important concept in pediatric nursing.
   A. Define family-centered care.

B. Indicate how you would go about providing this care.

2. Examine the graphs illustrating pediatric mortality statistics. Which populations are at highest risk for the following causes of death? What accounts for the higher rates in these age groups? (*Hint:* It may be helpful to review the information presented in Chapter 2.)
   A. Homicide
   B. Drowning
   C. Motor vehicle–related injuries
   D. Fires and burns

3. List three advantages of home care for chronically ill children.

4. What must be documented in a patient's record?

5. When may minor children give informed consent?

Critical Thinking: Application/Analysis

MULTIPLE CHOICE

Select the best answer.

1. Many more children with chronic conditions are now attending school since the enactment of the Education for All Handicapped Children Act because:

   A. All school nurses must now be registered nurses
   B. Care provided in schools is more cost effective than that in institutions
   C. Needed medical care must be available in school
   D. Schools must now have ramps and elevators for easy access

2. Incorporating a family's cultural beliefs into a plan of care is vital because it facilitates:

   A. Nursing staff's understanding of the family's beliefs
   B. Parents' ability to direct their child's care
   C. Family's compliance with care needed for their child
   D. Family's comfort in the hospital setting

3. The pediatric nurse best uses morbidity and mortality statistics when:

   A. Giving anticipatory guidance to patients and parents
   B. Planning care of hospitalized children
   C. Preparing standardized nursing care plans
   D. Anticipating the needs of hospitalized children

4. Which of the following has had a positive impact on the cost of health care?

   A. Development of lifesaving technologies
   B. Decrease in hospital admissions
   C. Insurance coverage for all children
   D. Home care services paid for by federal funds

5. You are obtaining parents' signatures on a consent form for their child's surgery when one of the parents asks about complications that could arise from the surgery. You would:

   A. Answer the question to the best of your ability.
   B. Assure the parents that complications rarely occur, so it is not necessary to know every detail.
   C. Inform the child's physician that the parents still have questions.
   D. Have the parents sign the consent form, since you are only witnessing the signature.

6. When a nurse is teaching a child, the most important consideration is:

   A. To avoid frightening the child
   B. Child's developmental level
   C. Child's attention span
   D. Parental approval of content

7. Educating parents in the care of their children is an important nursing role because parents:

   A. Are often uncomfortable in the hospital setting
   B. Are the best persons to support their children
   C. Need to follow the hospital routines
   D. Can then teach their children

CASE STUDIES

1. Five-year old Yasmeen is diagnosed with insulin-dependent diabetes mellitus. The therapeutic regimen includes dietary restrictions and daily insulin injections.
   A. What are some cultural issues and family beliefs that can have a negative impact on the health care of this child at home?
   B. How can these issues and beliefs be addressed in the hospital setting?

2. The parents of Joel, who is 12 years old and has leukemia, refuse to allow anyone to discuss his illness and possible treatment with him. Their rationale is that he is too young and this information would only upset him. Based on your knowledge of growth and development, as well as informed consent, how would you approach his parents?

3. Three-week-old Tran was admitted with dehydration following 12 hours of diarrhea. His family is from Cambodia. Upon admission, an IV was started in Tran's hand. When his family went home overnight, Tran was resting comfortably. Later, the IV infiltrated and could only be restarted using a scalp vein. In the morning, the family returned and became very upset about the IV location and threatened to take Tran home. What may be the cause of their distress and how could it have been avoided?

Suggested Learning Activities

1. Using institutional standards of care, nurses regularly review the care given to their patients. When a trend of noncompliance is found, the problem must be identified. A plan of action is implemented and the standard is reevaluated to determine whether the problem has been resolved. This is the process of quality assurance; its goal is to improve nursing care. Apply this process to the following scenario. An increase in the readmission of children with asthma has been identified. A quality assurance study is planned and implemented to study this trend.

A. What factors influencing this trend might be identified?

B. What actions might be taken to resolve the problem?

2. Every hospital has an ethics committee. Select and interview a member of an ethics committee. Some possible questions and issues to explore are:

A. Who are the members of the committee, and what disciplines do they represent?

B. What are some of the recent decisions made by the committee?

C. Is there a standard process used by the committee to make decisions?

D. How would this exercise benefit you in your nursing practice?

3. Obtain a copy of the Nurse Practice Act for the state in which you will be licensed. What are the legal roles and responsibilities of nurses practicing in your state?

4. Review several critical pathways currently in use. How many departments are involved in these comprehensive interdisciplinary care plans? Are the sequence and timing of interventions logical and appropriate? How are these pathways an improvement over the previous care plans that were written and executed only by nurses?

5. Select an ethnic group that is different from your own. Research various aspects of this group—religion, health beliefs, social beliefs, roles and influence of various family members, and child-rearing practices. If a child from this ethnic group were admitted to the hospital, what information would be essential for the health care team to give culturally sensitive care to this child and family?

Answers with Rationales

Review of Concepts

Matching

1.

1. C	2. A	3. D
4. B	5. C	6. A
7. C	8. B	9. D

2.

1. C	2. I	3. E
4. B	5. H	6. A
7. D	8. F	9. G

Short Essay

1. A. Integration of the family's values and potential contributions into the planning and implementation of the child's care.

   B. Assess the family's cultural beliefs and values, as well as their response to the child's current and past illnesses. Next, plan care that incorporates the family's input. Implement the plan, encouraging parental participation as appropriate and supporting the family in their care and decisionmaking. Finally, prepare the family for discharge so that they can assume full responsibility for care after their child leaves the hospital.

2. Populations at high risk:
   A. *Homicide:*
      1–12 months—child abuse
      15–19 years—murder by other teens and adults
   B. *Drowning:*
      1–4 years—top-heavy and unable to swim
      15–19 years—risk taking
   C. *Motor vehicle–related injuries:*
      1–9 years—no seat belt, running into road, bike/car collision
   D. *Fires and burns:*
      1–4 years—playing with matches, unable to escape house fire

3. A. Parental control of care
   B. Lower cost
   C. Child participates in family and community

4. The following must be documented accurately and sequentially:
   A. Patient assessment
   B. Nursing care plan
   C. Child's response to medical therapies and nursing care
   D. Any untoward incidents that could inhibit patient's recovery
   E. Date, time, and nurse's signature and title

5. A. When they are parents of a child patient
   B. When they are emancipated minors
   C. When they are adolescents between 16 and 18 years of age seeking birth control, an abortion, mental health counseling, or substance abuse treatment (*Note:* State laws may differ on the definition of an emancipated minor; therefore it is necessary to determine the law in the state in which you will be practicing.)

Critical Thinking: Application/Analysis

Multiple Choice

1. C. The Education for All Handicapped Children Act provides free education to all handicapped children from 2 to 21 years of age. Because of this act, provisions for needed medical care must be available in the school setting.

2. C. If cultural values are not incorporated into the nursing care plan, conflicts can occur between the family's traditional practices and current health care practices, forcing families to choose between their traditions and compliance with the plan of care.

3. A. The factors placing children at high risk for unintentional death can be emphasized when giving guidance to parents and patients, possibly preventing an unnecessary death.

4. D. Home care financing with federal funds has dramatically decreased the cost of caring for chronically ill children who previously could be cared for only in hospitals or nursing homes.

5. C. Explanation of the risks of surgery is the physician's responsibility, and the parents should not sign a consent form until their questions have been answered.

6. B. The nurse needs to tailor teaching to the child's developmental level. A 5-year-old can understand very basic concrete information (e.g., "You will go into a big room and have a picture taken of your chest with a special camera"), whereas an adolescent is able to understand a complex explanation of an x-ray.

7. B. The child is influenced by and is dependent on the family. The parents know their child better than strangers do and their child will accept care from parents more readily than from strangers.

CASE STUDIES

1. A. Possible cultural issues:
   Dietary regimen: The family's diet may include ethnic food choices that can cause problems for management of the child's condition (e.g., diet high in concentrated sweets, vegetarian diet, pasta- or starch-based diet), or the timing of meals could place the child at risk (e.g., long interval between lunch and dinner).
   Insulin injections: Restriction against giving medications or injections.

   B. Methods of addressing issues in hospital setting:
   Diet: Assess the home diet and enlist the help of a nutritionist and the parents in planning a diet that the family can follow. For example, if late dinners are common, the child can adjust timing of snacks and afternoon insulin.
   Insulin injections: Teach the family about the purpose and action of insulin, and explain that there is no alternative treatment. If the family refuses to learn to administer insulin, refer them to a home health agency that can work with them in the home environment. (*Note:* If the family were to withhold the child's insulin, it could result in the child's death. This would be child neglect and the nurse would be required to report the action to Child Protective Services.)

2. By age 11, a child's abstract reasoning and logic are advanced. Both children and parents have the right to refuse treatment at any time; however, if this child is not told about the treatment, he cannot participate in the decision process.

3. The Cambodian culture has many beliefs that are different from those of people raised in America. One belief is that the head is where the person's luck or spirit resides, and it is bad luck if someone touches the head without permission. This case study demonstrates how lack of knowledge of a family's background can create severe distress for the family. This situation could have been avoided by asking the family about their cultural beliefs and taboos and keeping them informed of any changes that occurred in the care of the child. If there is a large immigrant population from one or two countries in a particular area, cultural research should be done on these populations to make future contacts by health care providers more positive.

GROWTH AND DEVELOPMENT

Chapter Overview

Chapter 2 focuses on the growth and development of children from infancy through adolescence. Principles of normal growth, influences on development, and major theories of development are discussed. In-depth discussions of each age group are presented, covering the topics of physical growth, cognitive development, play, nutrition, injury prevention, personality, temperament, and communication.

Learning Objectives

After studying this chapter, you should be able to:
- Describe the general principles of growth and development.
- Apply the theories of Piaget, Erikson, and Freud to children ranging in age from birth to adolescence.
- Identify physical and behavioral milestones that are characteristic of children in each age group.
- Recognize coping strategies used by children and adolescents.
- Describe normal patterns of play exhibited by children.
- List toys that are appropriate for young children.
- Discuss normal nutrition for children in each age group.
- Identify various hazards that can cause injuries to children and adolescents.
- Discuss characteristics of children's communication from birth through adolescence.

Review of Concepts

COMPLETION

1. Toddlers are at high risk for injuries because of their increasing cognitive and motor skills and curiosity. List measures that could prevent injury from the following hazards.

Hazard	Preventive Measures
A. Falls	
B. Poisoning	
C. Burns	
D. Motor vehicle crashes	
E. Drowning	

2. Adolescents are at high risk for injuries because of their increased independence. List measures that could prevent injuries from the following hazards.

Hazard	Preventive Measures
A. Motor vehicle crashes	
B. Sporting injuries	
C. Drowning	

MATCHING

Match the items in list 1 with the appropriate word or definition in list 2. (*Note:* Items may be used more than once.)

1. Developmental Milestones

LIST 1
A. Infant
B. Toddler
C. Preschool child
D. School-age child
E. Adolescent

LIST 2
1. ____ Frequent temper tantrums
2. ____ Rebellion against parents
3. ____ Likes collections
4. ____ Likes pull toys
5. ____ Triples weight in 12 months
6. ____ Brushes teeth
7. ____ Learns to tie shoes
8. ____ Rides bicycle
9. ____ At risk for choking
10. ____ Uses pincer grasp

2. Developmental Theories

LIST 1
A. Erikson
B. Freud
C. Bronfenbrenner
D. Piaget
E. Kohlberg
F. Bandura
G. Watson
H. Chess and Thomas

LIST 2
1. Psychosexual development
2. Cognitive development
3. Moral development
4. Temperament theory
5. Psychosocial development
6. Behaviorism
7. Ecologic theory
8. Social learning theory

SHORT ESSAY

1. List five reasons why knowledge of growth and development is necessary for pediatric nursing.

2. Every child is born with a certain genetic potential for growth and development. List five factors in the environment that can adversely affect this potential.

3. The behavior of a hospitalized child demonstrates regression to an earlier stage of development. How would you explain this behavior to the parents?

4. Discuss several strategies to help a 9-year-old child cope with hospitalization.

5. Describe the characteristics of adolescents that place them at greater risk for injuries.

Critical Thinking: Application/Analysis

MULTIPLE CHOICE

Select the best answer.

1. Which of the following examples demonstrates the principle of cephalocaudal development?

   A. Toddler can scribble before drawing a circle.
   B. Infant uses whole hand to pick up object before using finger and thumb.
   C. Infant is able to crawl before walking.
   D. Toddler throws ball, whereas preschooler gently rolls it.

2. The parents of a 4-year-old boy are worried because he often touches his genitals. The nurse's best response is to:

   A. Tell parents to slap child's hand whenever he is observed touching his genitals.
   B. Formulate a behavior modification program to decrease frequency of masturbation.
   C. Explain that this is normal behavior and that child should not be punished.
   D. Tell parents to quickly remove child's hand whenever he is observed masturbating.

3. A child denies that he has wet the bed. This is an example of the defense mechanism of:

   A. Repression
   B. Regression
   C. Rationalization
   D. Fantasy

4. A hospitalized toddler insists on drinking from a bottle even though she has been drinking regularly from a cup. This is an example of:

   A. Repression
   B. Regression
   C. Rationalization
   D. Fantasy

5. A toddler who has a temper tantrum is demonstrating:

   A. Shame
   B. Mistrust
   C. Autonomy
   D. Guilt

6. A 4-year-old child hospitalized with an unintentional injury may attribute the hospital admission to:

   A. Clumsiness
   B. Carelessness on playground
   C. Punishment for previous misdeeds
   D. Need to rest and get better

7. A 6-year-old child who is told to stop doing something becomes upset and angrily says to his mother, "You are lying." Although the mother tries to explain to the child why this is untrue, the child still insists that she is lying. This scenario illustrates the cognitive level of a preoperational child because at this stage:

   A. Language development is rapid
   B. Abstract concepts are not understood
   C. Child truly believes parent is lying
   D. Child is egocentric

8. A 4-month-old infant is able to:

   A. Turn head to look for sounds
   B. Turn from back to abdomen
   C. Sit without support
   D. Hold hand in fist

9. An 8-month-old infant is able to:

   A. Scribble with crayon
   B. Hold hand in fist
   C. Transfer object from one hand to other
   D. Stand alone

10. By 12 months of age, an infant characteristically:

    A. Uses fork and spoon well
    B. Plays peek-a-boo

C. Crawls with trunk on floor
D. Has quadrupled in birth weight

11. A problem with infant formulas that must be prepared is:

A. They are most expensive
B. They require sterile water for mixing
C. They can be mixed incorrectly
D. They are not as nutritious as other types

12. Following the eruption of teeth in an infant, the parent should be instructed to:

A. Brush infant's teeth daily and rinse with water
B. Avoid putting infant to bed with bottle of milk
C. Increase milk intake to keep calcium levels high
D. Stop breast-feeding to avoid nipple damage

13. Which of the following formulas can be given to a child with an allergy to milk?

A. SMA
B. Similac
C. Enfamil
D. Isomil

14. Which of the following toys would be appropriate for a 12-month-old infant?

A. Mobiles and books
B. Pull toys and blocks
C. Big Wheel tricycle and puzzles
D. Teething rings and rattles

15. It is recommended that rice cereal be introduced into the infant diet at 4 to 6 months of age because:

A. Infant needs to learn how to eat from spoon
B. Rice cereal is not tolerated at earlier age
C. Infant needs solid food to feel satisfied
D. Rice cereal is good source of iron

16. A new mother tells you that her 4-month-old infant keeps spitting out his cereal when she feeds him. Your best response would be to tell her:

A. "He is not ready for solid foods. Wait a few months and try again."

B. "He does not like the taste but will get used to it over time."
C. "This is a normal reflex. Carefully place food inside his mouth beyond the tip of the tongue."
D. "You are probably feeding him too much at a time. Give him smaller amounts."

17. Anticipatory guidance for mothers who are using prepared baby foods would be:

A. Avoid prepared combination foods such as vegetable-beef dinners
B. Buy only a 3-day supply because of short shelf-life
C. Feed infant more fruits than vegetables each day
D. Avoid giving meats to infant until 18 months of age

18. Infants are not fed honey in the first 12 months of life because:

A. Honey is high in concentrated sugars
B. They can develop botulism
C. They will be predisposed to obesity
D. All other foods that are not sweet will be refused

19. Older infants are at high risk for choking because:

A. They explore objects by placing them in mouth
B. They do not chew their food
C. Their suck and swallow reflexes are not coordinated
D. They forget to swallow because they are so busy

20. By 2 years of age, a child can:

A. Use fork and spoon well
B. Build tower of four blocks
C. Use scissors
D. Brush teeth

21. A type of play that is common in toddlers is:

A. Parallel play
B. Solitary play
C. Onlooker play
D. Interactive play

22. A mother tells you that she is concerned about her daughter's diet. The toddler eats smaller amounts of food and is not very interested in eating. Your best response would be to tell the mother:

A. "If this problem persists, you should see your child's doctor to get advice on a special diet."
B. "A toddler's stomach is small and can tolerate only small meals."
C. "Give her more milk and juices if she isn't interested in solids."
D. "This is a normal change. Toddlers are growing more slowly and don't need as much food."

23. Placing an adhesive bandage over an injection site is very important to a toddler because:

A. It helps prevent infection, since a toddler will rub and pick at site
B. This action allows a nurse time to soothe the toddler
C. Toddler may fear that his or her insides will leak out
D. This is a ritual that most toddlers perform at home

24. Temper tantrums are most common during toddlerhood because the child is:

A. Searching for independence
B. Unable to understand parents
C. Having difficulty with discipline
D. Easily exhausted from constant activity

25. While having blood drawn, a 5-year-old child screams, "Why are you hurting me? I haven't done anything wrong." This is an example of:

A. Guilt
B. Animism
C. Magical thinking
D. Egocentrism

26. The nurse can use puppets for therapeutic communication with a 5-year-old child because preschoolers:

A. Normally engage in dramatic play

B. Display animism with toys
C. Are able to manipulate the puppets
D. Are afraid to speak directly to adults

27. A 3-year-old child cries out that the CT scanning machine is going to eat her. This is an example of:

A. Dramatic play
B. Animisim
C. Egocentrism
D. Centration

28. When told that the nurse is going to take his pulse, a 4-year-old boy asks, "Will you give it back?" This is an example of:

A. Initiative
B. Humor
C. Animism
D. Preoperational thought

29. Preschool children are at highest risk for injury from:

A. Poisoning by ingesting medications
B. Falls from great heights
C. Motor vehicle–pedestrian crashes
D. Child abuse by parents and caretakers

30. School-age children are able to play baseball on a team. This is an example of:

A. Associative play
B. Cooperative play
C. Solitary play
D. Parallel play

31. A 9-year-old child demonstrates a sense of industry by:

A. Explaining workings of the heart
B. Running for short distances
C. Making a collection of several objects
D. Building with plastic blocks

32. Adolescents struggle with identity formation. A major challenge to their identity is:

A. Dramatic changes in their bodies

B. Development of abstract thought
C. Parent–child relationship
D. Relationships with younger children

33. Color blindness is a condition that is passed to children on the X chromosome. The chance that a man who is unaffected and a woman who is a carrier will have a son who is color blind is:

A. 0%
B. 25%
C. 50%
D. 100%

CASE STUDIES

1. The mother of a 2½-year-old child is very upset because the child is not yet toilet trained. What information about toilet training would you provide to allay her anxiety?

2. Eight-year-old John is constantly going to his friend's house to play for long periods of time and is seldom home. His mother is concerned because he seems to be avoiding his family, which, in the past, was very closely knit. What guidance about this behavior would you give to John's mother?

3. Mendelian Inheritance
   A. A man who is color blind is married to a woman who is a carrier for color blindness. What are the chances that any boys they have will be color blind and any girls will be carriers or color blind?
   B. A man who carries a recessive gene for sickle cell anemia is married to a woman who also carries the recessive gene for sickle cell anemia. What are the chances that their children will be carriers or have the disease?

Suggested Learning Activities

1. Contact the LaLeche League in your area. Investigate the services that are available to breast-feeding mothers while in the hospital and after discharge.

2. Arrange a visit to a day care center during an active play time. Observe two toddlers who are close in age. Analyze their activities and behaviors using the theories of Erikson, Freud, and Piaget.

3. Interview an adolescent who has recently been hospitalized. Areas to explore might include (1) what was most disturbing about the admission, (2) which experiences were expected and which were not expected, (3) whether friends and family were allowed to visit, and (4) what changes could be made to make the hospitalization experience more positive.

ANSWERS WITH RATIONALES

Review of Concepts

COMPLETION

1. Toddler

Hazard	Preventive Measures
A. Falls	Supervise closely. Teach acceptable places for climbing. Ensure that ladders are properly stored. Never leave ladder unattended in upright position.
B. Poisoning	Keep medicine and poisons in locked cabinet or out of reach. Use child-resistant containers appropriately. Keep number of poison control center by telephone. Keep syrup of ipecac in home (see Chapter 15).
C. Burns	Keep pot handles turned inward on stove. Prevent child from climbing up to stove and reaching for items on counters in kitchen. Supervise closely when near fire.
D. Motor vehicle crashes	Use approved safety seat whenever car is in motion. (Be adamant because child will resist use of safety seat.)
E. Drowning	Supervise child closely when near any water: pool, stream, bathtub, toilet, or bucket. (Toddlers are top-heavy and may not be able to get out of water if they fall in head-first.) Use life jackets when boating. Use child-resistant pool covers (see Chapter 11).

2. Adolescent

Hazard	Preventive Measures
A. Motor vehicle crashes	Insist on driver's education classes and use of seat belts. Enforce rules about safe driving. Discourage alcohol and drug use.
B. Sporting injuries	Encourage use of protective gear and proper warm-up. Have injuries evaluated by health care professionals. Discourage alcohol and drug use.
C. Drowning	Discourage swimming alone. Enforce rules of the swimming area. Inform about risks.

MATCHING

1.
1. B	2. E	3. D
4. A, B	5. A	6. C, D, E
7. C	8. D	9. A, B
10. A		

2.
1. B	2. D	3. E
4. H	5. A	6. G
7. C	8. F	

SHORT ESSAY

1. Knowledge of growth and development in children is necessary in order to:
   A. Identify areas of abnormal development.
   B. Guide nurse in planning interventions for child and family.
   C. Plan teaching approaches based on language and cognitive development of child.

D. Provide appropriate activities and toys during illness or hospitalization.

E. Respond therapeutically during interactions with child.

2. Possible answers include:
   A. *Prenatal influences* — maternal factors such as smoking, poor nutrition and health, ingestion of alcohol and drugs, acquired diseases (HIV infection, rubella), exposure to radiation, environmental hazards.
   B. *Family structure* — size and composition of family, birth order, divorce, single parenting, joint custody arrangements.
   C. *Stress* — stressful events for children include moving to a new home or school, marital difficulties in family, abuse, being expected to achieve at an extremely high level.
   D. *Socioeconomic influences* — poverty, poor nutrition, homelessness.
   E. *Community* — high homicide rate in community, contaminated water supplies, crowded living conditions, air pollution.
   F. *Culture* — traditional foods that could compromise health, rules regarding patterns of social interaction (e.g., rigid gender roles).
   G. *Media* — violence on television and games associated with aggressive behavior.

3. Regression is a common defense mechanism used by children to protect themselves from excess anxiety. Once the child returns home to a normal routine and feels less threatened, the regressive behavior will disappear.

4. The 9-year-old is in the stage of industry vs. inferiority, when it is important to the child to accomplish good work. A sense of achievement derived from accomplishments is important in the development of self-worth. Because rules are important at this age, the hospitalized child needs to understand the hospital and unit rules. The 9-year-old child is able to understand explanations of tests and disease cognitively; however, concrete examples and materials are necessary for greater understanding. Because separation from friends is difficult for school-age children, visits by friends are encouraged. If possible, the child should be placed with a roommate who is close to the child's age. The child can be encouraged to continue with many quiet activities normally engaged in at home (e.g., hobbies, collections, reading, puzzles). The school-age child may be resistant to new foods in the hospital, so parents should be encouraged to bring in foods from home, if appropriate.

5. Adolescents often feel invulnerable. Because they feel that no harm can come to them, they engage in many dangerous behaviors. They also have easy access to potentially harmful objects such as guns, cars, drugs, and alcohol.

Critical Thinking: Application/Analysis

MULTIPLE CHOICE

1. C. Cephalocaudal development proceeds from the head to the tail.

2. C. Preschoolers are in Freud's phallic stage of development. Masturbation by the young child is normal.

3. A. Repression is the forgetting of painful experiences or uncomfortable situations.

4. B. Regression involves a return to an earlier behavior in response to a threat or anxiety.

5. C. The toddler shows autonomy by saying no when asked to do something or by having a tantrum when told not to do something.

6. C. According to Piaget, a 4-year-old child relies on transductive reasoning (drawing conclusions from one general fact to another). An example of this is magical thinking. Because the cause-and-effect relationship is unrealistic, the child may attribute an injury or illness to some previous unrelated behavior, believing the illness or injury to be punishment for that "bad" behavior.

7. B. In the preoperational stage, language skills blossom. Logic is not well developed, however, and the child is unable to use abstract terms and reasoning. "Lying" is a common word, but its meaning is abstract and therefore not well understood by the child in this stage of development.

8. A. A 4-month-old infant has developed some control of the neck muscles and can actively move the head from side to side to locate sound.

9. C. Development progresses in the proximodistal direction. By 8 months, the infant is able to use the whole hand to grasp an object; by 10 months, he or she progresses to the ability to pick up an object with the thumb and forefinger (pincer grasp).

10. B. Infants engage in peek-a-boo once they have attained the concept of object permanence. The 12-month-old infant understands that when a face is covered it still exists and can be seen again.

11. C. A powder or liquid formula that is not diluted properly places the infant at nutritional risk. When the formula is too concentrated, the infant may be at risk for hypernatremia (see Chapter 8). When the formula is too dilute, the infant receives too few calories. When assessing an infant's nutritional status, always ask parents what formula they use and how it is prepared.

12. B. Milk pools in the mouth as the infant falls asleep. This causes a decrease in salivary flow, which decreases acid buffering and results in tooth decay. Tooth decay can be so severe that the baby teeth need to be capped to enable the child to chew food.

13. D. Isomil is a soy-based formula. Since soy formulas have no milk content, they are usually tolerated well by infants with milk allergies. (See Chapter 15 for further discussion of cow's milk sensitivity.)

14. B. A 12-month-old infant is beginning to walk and move about. A pull toy makes walking more interesting, encouraging the infant to practice this skill. The infant is also able to hold and manipulate blocks.

15. D. Rice cereal is an easily digested source of iron and has low allergenic potential. Iron intake is important at 4 to 6 months of age because prenatal iron stores have become depleted and need to be replaced.

16. C. Young infants have a protrusion reflex or tongue thrust that makes it difficult to give solids with a spoon. Placement of a small spoonful on the top of the tongue inside the mouth helps to minimize the "spitting out" of food.

17. A. Combination meals and desserts usually contain more sugar, salt, and fillers. "Dinners" are usually very light on meats and heavy on fillers and vegetables.

18. B. Honey is not sterilized and can contain *Clostridium botulinum* spores. Infants are unable to detoxify these spores and may develop botulism. Some people dip pacifiers in honey to soothe a fretful baby. Parents need to be cautioned against this practice.

19. A. Objects are placed in the mouth because the infant derives pleasure from sucking and eating (see discussion about Freud). Small toys or hard foods such as nuts and hot dogs can easily cause choking.

20. B. As development of fine motor skills progresses, the child has more control of the hands and can stack four blocks. The ability to use a fork and spoon well, use scissors, and brush teeth is characteristic of older children.

21. A. Toddlers tend to play side by side with similar objects, but not with each other. For example, two toddlers who are playing with blocks will build only their own creations, not a common structure.

22. D. During infancy, the metabolic needs are very high because of the rapid growth that occurs

(the infant triples his or her birth weight in 12 months). The growth rate slows dramatically in the second year of life, reducing the child's need for a large intake of food. This response is called physiologic anorexia. The child's intake should be recorded over several days to obtain an accurate assessment of nutritional intake. Food should be offered in small amounts several times a day, and milk should be decreased to 16 to 24 ounces a day.

23. C. The toddler is developing a sense of control over his or her body and is unable to comprehend what would happen if a hole is made in the skin.

24. A. The toddler is striving for autonomy or independence. When told to do something, the toddler often has a tantrum because he or she is not in control of the situation. The tantrum is a form of communication, not "bad" behavior. However, it is upsetting to parents. Parents can be taught the following strategies to deal with a tantrum: (1) acknowledge why the child is angry, (2) state that when the child stops crying he or she can return to the family area, and (3) ignore all further negative behavior.

25. C. Magical thinking is a form of transductive reasoning in which the child connects two unrelated events in a cause-and-effect relationship. Preschoolers may believe that a negative or painful procedure is punishment for a previous misdeed.

26. A. Preschoolers engage in dramatic play in which they live out the drama of human life. The nurse can use this approach when explaining procedures or evaluating the child's knowledge of illness.

27. B. Animism is a characteristic of preoperational thought in which the preschooler gives lifelike qualities to nonliving things. A CT scanner has a large hole in the center into which the child's body is placed for the examination. To the preschooler, this hole resembles a large mouth. The nurse needs to anticipate this fear and discuss what the machine looks like and what will happen before the procedure is begun.

28. D. In preoperational thought, words are used as symbols, but the child's grasp of meaning is usually literal and logic is not well developed. The child interprets the reference to taking something to mean that it will be removed from the body.

29. C. Preschoolers are becoming more independent and mobile. They are unable to judge the speed of an approaching car and assume that the driver can see them.

30. B. Cooperative play requires cooperation with others and the ability to play a part in order to contribute to a unified whole.

31. C. Collections and hobbies are two of the favorite play activities of school-age children. Both activities promote a sense of industry, which is important to the child at this developmental stage.

32. A. During adolescence, the body undergoes rapid physical and hormonal changes that take place over a period of several years. As each change occurs, there is a corresponding change in identity.

33. C. In each pregnancy resulting in a male child, when the father is not color blind and the mother is a carrier for color blindness, the child has a 50% chance of being color blind and a 50% chance of being unaffected. If the woman is pregnant with a girl, the chance of the girl being a carrier is 50% and of being unaffected is 50%. Females have more protection from this genetic disorder because all females have two X chromosomes. When a woman is a carrier, the second X chromosome prevents the color blindness from being manifested, but she can pass the disorder on to her children.

CASE STUDIES

1. Children are not able to be toilet trained until the following developmental milestones have been achieved: (1) the ability to stand and walk well, (2) the ability to pull pants up and down, (3) the ability to recognize the need to urinate or defecate, and (4) the ability to wait to urinate or defecate until in the bathroom. If any of these abilities is not present, training will probably be unsuccessful. Training occurs with considerable variability from one child to another and is not predictive of future development.

2. The school-age child enjoys spending time with others of the same age. Cooperative play, in which the child works with others to accomplish a goal, is a hallmark of this age group. Spending more time with peers is part of the social component of play. The nurse needs to emphasize the importance of this behavior in the child's normal development.

3. Mendelian Inheritance
   A. This case study is an example of X-linked inheritance. A man who is color blind will pass on the X chromosome with the color blindness gene on it to all of his daughters. The woman who is a carrier will pass on the X chromosome with the color blindness gene to 50% of her daughters. Therefore, the daughters from these parents will be 50% carriers and 50% color blind (both X chromosomes have the color blindness gene; therefore, the girl will be color blind). In the case of the sons, the man will not pass on his color blindness gene to his sons so the chance of his sons being color blind is 50%.

   B. This case study is an example of recessive inheritance in which both parents must have the gene for the disease or trait to be manifested in one of their children. When both parents carry the recessive gene for sickle cell anemia, 25% of their children will not carry the gene, 50% will be carriers, and 25% will have sickle cell anemia. Because the disease can only be manifested when both parents are carriers, the diagnosis of the disorder in a child can be a great shock to a family that was unaware that they carried the genes for the disease.

PEDIATRIC ASSESSMENT

Chapter Overview

Chapter 3 focuses on the assessment of children. Areas of emphasis include obtaining an appropriate history and performing a complete physical examination. Each body system is discussed in detail, outlining the normal and abnormal findings that may be noted.

Learning Objectives

After studying this chapter, you should be able to:
- Obtain a thorough history, including patient information, physiologic data, and psychosocial data.
- Describe strategies to increase the cooperation of children during the physical examination.
- Select appropriate assessment techniques for each body system being examined.
- Describe normal and abnormal findings for each body system.
- Discuss the normal sequence of development found in boys and girls during puberty.
- Distinguish among the primitive reflexes found in infants.

Review of Concepts

COMPLETION

1. Primitive Reflexes

Reflex	Appearance	Disappearance
A. Babinski		
B. Moro		
C. Palmar grasp		
D. Plantar grasp		
E. Stepping		
F. Tonic neck		
G. Placing		

List 2
1. _____ Mouth
2. _____ Chest
3. _____ Ear
4. _____ Head
5. _____ Abdomen

MATCHING

Match the items in list 1 with the appropriate word or phrase in list 2. (*Note:* Items may be used more than once.)

1. Inspection of Skin

List 1
A. Normal skin variation
B. Abnormal skin variation

List 2
1. _____ Bruise
2. _____ Freckles
3. _____ Jaundice
4. _____ Skin tenting
5. _____ Mongolian spot
6. _____ Papule

2. Normal Heart Rates

List 1
A. 60
B. 80
C. 100
D. 120
E. 140
F. 160

List 2
1. _____ Newborn
2. _____ Infants to 2 years
3. _____ 2–6 years
4. _____ 6–10 years
5. _____ 10–16 years

3. Assessment Techniques

Select appropriate techniques for each area of the body being examined.

List 1
A. Inspection
B. Palpation
C. Percussion
D. Auscultation

SHORT ESSAY

1. Discuss cultural issues that must be considered when obtaining a child's history.

2. The mother of a young girl is questioning when her daughter will begin to "develop" and what she should expect. What guidance would you give her?

3. Physical examination of a toddler can be difficult. Describe three factors that can be barriers and the strategies you would use to overcome them.

Critical Thinking: Application/Analysis

MULTIPLE CHOICE

Select the best answer.

1. Infants with Mongolian spots:

   A. Will have pain until spots fade
   B. Are often anemic and require iron supplements
   C. May be misidentified as victims of abuse
   D. Are treated with skin grafting

2. Scalp hair loss on a child may be due to:

   A. Premature balding
   B. Tight braiding of hair
   C. Allergy to medications
   D. Head lice

3. The anterior fontanel normally closes between:

   A. 20–30 months of age
   B. 6–10 months of age

C. 12–18 months of age

D. 2–3 months of age

4. The corneal light reflex is a simple test for:

   A. Glaucoma
   B. Cataracts
   C. Visual acuity
   D. Strabismus

5. A simple test of an infant's vision involves:

   A. Shining light in eye and watching pupil constrict
   B. Observing infant as he or she watches mother's face
   C. Moving object from side to side to see if infant follows with eyes
   D. Performing a cover-uncover test

6. To inspect the auditory canal of a 2-year-old child, it is necessary to pull the pinna:

   A. Up and back
   B. Up only
   C. Down and back
   D. Down only

7. At what point in the physical examination of a toddler should the tympanic membrane be examined?

   A. At beginning of examination
   B. Near end of examination
   C. When examining head and neck
   D. Before listening to chest sounds

8. An absent light reflex on the tympanic membrane is an indication of:

   A. Middle ear infection
   B. Retracted eardrum
   C. Perforated eardrum
   D. Blood in middle ear

9. Which of the following behaviors is an indication of hearing loss in a 6-month-old infant?

   A. Continued babbling
   B. No response to interesting sounds

C. Failure to speak first words
D. Absence of Moro reflex

10. A simple test for both air and bone conduction of sound is:

    A. Tap on forehead
    B. Weber test
    C. Rinne test
    D. Snellen test

11. Inspection of an infant's mouth reveals white adherent patches on the tongue and inner cheeks. The examiner correctly identifies this as a:

    A. Normal finding in infants
    B. Coating of formula
    C. *Candida* infection
    D. Geographic tongue

12. An infant's respirations should be counted for:

    A. 10 seconds and multiplied by 6
    B. 15 seconds and multiplied by 4
    C. 30 seconds and multiplied by 2
    D. 60 seconds

13. Which of the following is an abnormal finding when palpating the chest?

    A. Feeling heart beats
    B. Vocal resonance
    C. Tactile fremitus
    D. Crepitus

14. Auscultation of the chest of infants and young children is difficult because:

    A. Infants and young children breathe very shallowly
    B. Sounds in one lung are heard over entire area
    C. Ribs are closer together so sound is not heard as easily
    D. Stethoscopes are designed to be used for adults and are too large

15. A normal development at puberty that is often very distressing to boys is:

A. Breast buds
B. Leg hair
C. Body odor
D. Voice changes

16. Sinus arrhythmia is heard when auscultating the heart in a child. This finding is:

    A. Response to oxygen need
    B. Normal in children
    C. Murmur that should be reported
    D. Sign of congestive heart failure

17. The percussion tone of tympany is found in the abdomen over:

    A. Liver
    B. Stomach
    C. Kidneys
    D. Bladder

18. Which of the following strategies would facilitate palpation of a ticklish child's abdomen?

    A. Have child place his or her hand on abdomen with examiner's hand on top, fingers extending to skin
    B. Have examiner press hard on skin so tickling sensation is absent.
    C. Distract child with other sounds and tasks while touching abdomen.
    D. Place small amount of lubricant on skin so examiner's fingers slide easily.

19. A test to detect a congenital hip dislocation in a newborn is:

    A. Gower sign
    B. Heel-to-shin test
    C. Ortolani–Barlow maneuver
    D. Cremasteric reflex

20. A child's height and weight are plotted on a standardized growth chart. The results are 75th percentile for height and 25th percentile for weight. These findings would indicate that the child is:

    A. Underweight for height
    B. Overweight for height
    C. Tall
    D. Underweight

21. A child of Southeast Asian descent is measured, and the height and weight on the growth chart are both on the 10th percentile line. This should be interpreted as:

    A. Inadequate nutrition
    B. Normal growth
    C. Potential growth disorder
    D. Failure to thrive

CASE STUDIES

1. Sixteen-year-old Sara is admitted to the hospital following a car accident in which she was the driver. What psychosocial information should be obtained during her admission history?

2. You are preparing to do a physical assessment on a 14-year-old boy. His mother is sitting at his bedside. When you ask her to step out of the room, she becomes angry, telling you that she has always stayed with her son so that she can answer any questions that come up. How would you approach this mother about her presence during the examination?

Suggested Learning Activities

1. Perform a complete physical assessment on an infant, toddler, or school-age child. Record your results and compare them to the norms for that age group.

ANSWERS WITH RATIONALES

Review of Concepts

1. Primitive Reflexes

Reflex	Appearance	Disappearance
A. Babinski	Birth	2 years
B. Moro	Birth	6 months
C. Palmar grasp	Birth	3 months
D. Plantar grasp	Birth	8 months
E. Stepping	Birth	4 to 8 weeks
F. Tonic neck	2 months	6 months
G. Placing	Soon after birth	Various times

MATCHING

1.
1. B	2. A	3. B
4. B	5. A	6. B

2.
1. C, D, E, F	2. B, C, D	3. B, C, D
4. B, C	5. A, B, C	

3.
1. A, B	2. A, B, C, D	3. A
4. A, B	5. A, B, C, D	

SHORT ESSAY

1. Care must be taken to be certain that the child and parents understand the interviewer. The family may have a limited knowledge of English, and an interpreter may be necessary. Be certain the interpreter understands medical terms and is familiar with the cultural norms of the family. To protect the family's confidentiality, it is best to avoid having a family member or close friend act as an interpreter. Direct all communication to the parent or child, not the interpreter, during the interview. A basic knowledge of common cultural customs of people in the community is necessary. For example, some cultural groups avoid eye contact because it is deemed impolite or a sign of disrespect.

2. The first pubertal change experienced by girls is breast development, which normally occurs between 10 and 14 years of age. The first stage is budding, in which a bud-shaped elevation is noted. Initially, the breasts may be asymmetrical, which can be distressing to the child; however, this asymmetry usually resolves. The next change is the development of public hair, beginning with soft, downy hair along the labia majora. As development proceeds, the breasts continue to enlarge and assume the adult contour, and the pubic hair becomes more coarse and curly and spreads laterally. Approximately 2 years after breast bud development, menstruation begins. Any pubertal development before 8 years of age is abnormal.

3. Barriers to examining toddlers include stranger anxiety, egocentrism, and the toddler's limited ability to understand verbal communication. The following strategies could be used: Avoid touching the child initially. Allow the child to sit in the parent's lap while you talk first with the parent. This lets the child see that you are not a threat. Have the parent undress the child to the waist. Begin the examination by touching only the child's fingers and toes, and work toward the center of the body slowly. Talk to the child in simple language, using the child's perceptions as the basis of conversation. Trust is

demonstrated when the child begins to talk more readily to the examiner and touches the equipment. You can then proceed to examine the rest of the child's body.

Critical Thinking: Application/Analysis

Multiple Choice

1. C. Mongolian spots are large patches of bluish skin that are usually located on the buttocks, although they may be present anywhere on the body. They are a normal occurrence in dark-skinned infants; however, they can be mistaken for bruises from a spanking. The spots, which do not change color as a bruise would, should be well documented in the record in case any question arises in the future. Mongolian spots usually fade within the first few years of life.

2. B. Many cultures braid the hair of young children to keep it neat and tangle-free. When the hair is braided tightly, the tension can cause the hair to fall out, resulting in bald patches on the head.

3. C. The anterior fontanel becomes progressively smaller beginning at 6 months; it usually closes between 12 and 18 months of age. The posterior fontanel closes between 2 and 3 months of age.

4. D. The corneal light reflex is tested to detect the presence of a muscle imbalance that can result in strabismus. A light positioned in the center of the face and shining on the nose is reflected on the cornea of each eye. The reflection should be seen in the same area on each cornea. If not, strabismus should be suspected.

5. C. A young infant will follow an object moved slowly from side to side. Be certain that no sound accompanies the movement.

6. C. In children under 3 years of age, the auditory canal curves upward. To view the tympanic membrane, the canal must be straightened by moving the pinna downward and backward.

7. B. Infants and children often resist examination of the ear because of prior painful experiences or the need for restraint. Perform uncomfortable portions of the examination at the end, when further cooperation is not needed. Steps of the examination that require calm or cooperation, such as auscultating lungs, should be performed first.

8. A. An infection in the middle ear causes increased pressure behind the tympanic membrane. The light reflex from the otoscope light is not visible in a bulging eardrum.

9. B. A 6-month-old infant is expected to babble and make sounds. However, the infant also should be interested in locating other sounds.

10. C. The Rinne test is used to evaluate both air and bone conduction of sound. Air-conducted sound should be heard twice as long as bone-conducted sound.

11. C. *Candida* infection (thrush) is common in infants, particularly in the first few months of age or after treatment with antibiotics. Suspect thrush if the infant is pushing the nipple out of the mouth or is fussy during feedings. Although thrush can also occur in older children after antibiotic therapy, it is not as common.

12. D. Young infants normally have an irregular respiration rate. Therefore, the respirations should be counted for a full minute for accuracy.

13. D. Crepitus in any part of the chest may indicate a leak of air from the lungs into the tissues of the chest cavity or a fractured rib. Any finding of crepitus should be reported immediately.

14. B. The chest wall is thin because muscle development is immature. Sounds in one area are heard throughout the small chest. This makes it difficult to identify absent or abnormal sounds in different parts of the chest.

15. A. Boys often have unilateral or bilateral breast enlargement during adolescence. This enlarge-

ment can range from breast buds to actual breast tissue. This change normally disappears within a year.

16. B. Sinus arrhythmia is a normal cycle of irregular heart rhythms in children. The child's heart rate is faster on inspiration and slower on expiration. If the child takes a breath and holds it, the rhythm should become regular.

17. B. Tympany is the tone that results from vibration over an air-filled stomach.

18. A. The child feels more in control when his or her own hand is on the abdomen. Having the child place his or her hand on top of the examiner's hand is another possible approach.

19. C. The Ortolani–Barlow maneuver reveals a subluxation or dislocation of the hip. Subluxation is present when the head of the femur slips out of the hip joint. Dislocation is present when there is resistance to hip abduction.

20. A. When results on a growth chart are being examined, the height and weight must be compared. In this case, the child is tall for age, but also underweight for that height.

21. B. Many cultural groups were not included in the research that was used to establish the growth chart standards. The normal stature of children from these groups may be significantly lower or higher than the North American norms. A quick way to assess whether a child's growth results are normal is to look at the parents. If both are very tall or very short, their children will likely follow the same pattern. Multiple measurements taken over time illustrate the child's growth pattern. They should follow a curve that is similar to the shape of the norms. Some children may be far above or far below the norms but still be developing normally. (Refer to Chapter 20 for discussion of abnormal growth patterns and to Chapter 22 for failure to thrive.)

CASE STUDIES

1. Critical areas that should be discussed in the psychosocial history for adolescents include their home environment (Do you live at home? How do you get along with parents?), employment and education (Currently in school? Grades? Employment plans? Have you ever been expelled?), activities (What do you do for fun? Who do you spend time with?), drugs (Have you tried drugs or alcohol? Do you smoke or chew tobacco? Are your friends drug users or sellers?), sexual activity/sexuality (Are you sexually active? When did you start having sex? Do you use precautions? Have you ever been abused physically or sexually?), suicide/depression (Are you ever sad, tired, or unmotivated? Have you ever felt life is not worth living?), and safety (Do you use seat belts? Bike helmets? Is there a gun in your house?).

2. This patient is an adolescent who has the right to privacy and confidentiality. You should ask the mother to speak with you away from the child. The mother needs to understand her son's developmental need for privacy. Assure her that you will meet with her after the examination to address any of her concerns and to ask any quesetions that are still unanswered. When you are performing the examination, reassure the patient that the findings are confidential and that your discussion will not be repeated to his mother. This assurance should help him to be more open with his responses, particularly regarding his sexual history.

Nursing Considerations for the Hospitalized Child

Chapter Overview

Chapter 4 focuses on the adaptation of children and families to hospitalization. Strategies to decrease fear and anxiety in both the child and family are presented in detail. Preparation for procedures, surgery, long-term care, and rehabilitation are also addressed.

Learning Objectives

After studying this chapter, you should be able to:
- Describe children's understanding of health and illness from infancy through adolescence.
- Identify strategies to minimize separation anxiety in young children.
- Discuss strategies to decrease a child's fear of admission to the hospital.
- Discuss the stressors on the family when a child is admitted to the hospital.
- Describe the family's role in helping a child adapt to hospitalization.
- Identify strategies to promote coping and normal development during a child's hospitalization.
- Describe age-appropriate therapeutic play techniques.
- Describe how and when to prepare children for medical procedures.
- Outline a care plan for a child undergoing surgery.

Review of Concepts

MATCHING

Match the items in list 1 with the appropriate word or phrase in list 2. (*Note:* Items may be used more than once.)

1. Therapeutic Play Techniques

LIST 1
A. Toddler
B. Preschool child
C. School-age child

LIST 2
1. ____ Playing with equipment
2. ____ Crafts
3. ____ Dramatic play
4. ____ Drawing
5. ____ Reading to child
6. ____ Video games

Short Essay

1. Outline several strategies that parents can employ to improve their hospitalized child's coping ability when they are away from the hospital.

2. Describe several ways to prepare a child for an elective admission to the hospital.

3. Outline the assessment information that should be obtained about the family of a hospitalized child.

4. List strategies that may help children adapt to the hospital environment.

5. List preoperative interventions that might help a 4-year-old child learn about postoperative events.

Critical Thinking: Application/Analysis

Multiple Choice

Select the best answer.

1. When asked why he is in the hospital, a 3-year-old child responds, "I didn't share my candy with my sister, and that's why my stomach hurts." This is an example of:

   A. Magical thinking
   B. Animism
   C. Egocentrism
   D. Concrete thinking

2. A hospitalized 11-month-old infant begins to cry loudly when her parents prepare to leave the room. The stage of separation anxiety demonstrated is:

   A. Detachment
   B. Despair
   C. Protest
   D. Denial

3. A strategy to decrease the stress of hospitalization for a teenager is to:

   A. Keep curtains pulled to protect privacy
   B. Encourage parental presence all day
   C. Discourage friends from visiting
   D. Encourage peer visitation

4. Siblings of a hospitalized child can be affected negatively by their brother's or sister's hospitalization. To decrease this impact, parents might be advised to:

   A. Take them to visit their sibling if possible
   B. Send them to stay with other family members
   C. Stay home with them
   D. Avoid discussing hospitalized sibling

5. The parent of a hospitalized child has been taught how to perform a procedure. The next day, the parent asks several questions that were covered the day before. This most likely indicates that the parent:

   A. Is probably unable to understand information being presented
   B. Did not pay attention during initial teaching session
   C. Is not interested in performing procedure
   D. Was preoccupied and stressed during teaching session

6. When developing a teaching plan for a child, the nurse must:

   A. Consider child's level of development
   B. Be sure parents are present
   C. Ask parents to leave room
   D. Protect child from added stress

7. An effective therapeutic play technique for toddlers is to:

   A. Have them draw pictures of their fears
   B. Repeatedly read familiar stories
   C. Involve them in dramatic play with dolls
   D. Have them make up a story from a picture

8. The most effective strategy to help adolescents cope with hospitalization is to:

   A. Give them a book about their illness

B. Have them draw pictures about their experiences
C. Invite their friends to visit and watch a movie
D. Encourage them to play with younger patients

9. Painful procedures should be performed on toddlers and preschoolers in a treatment room because:

A. Child's crying will be less disruptive to other patients
B. Child's room and bed must remain a safe haven
C. All necessary equipment is nearby
D. Lighting and layout are better in treatment room

10. Discharge planning should begin:

A. 24 hours before discharge
B. On admission
C. At time of discharge
D. Once patient's condition is stabilized

11. The Gellert Index assesses a child's:

A. Knowledge of body
B. Level of comfort
C. Pain level
D. Cognitive level

CASE STUDIES

1. Nine-year-old Jerome will be undergoing insertion of a tibial traction pin within the next 24 hours. Describe how and when you would prepare this child for the painful invasive procedure.

2. A 4-year-old girl is being treated for peritonitis following the rupture of her appendix. She is receiving intravenous antibiotics and requires frequent site changes. In addition, her surgical incision is open and requires packing each shift. The child is fearful and cries whenever staff members approach her bed. To reduce her fear and stress, what therapeutic play techniques would you implement?

Suggested Learning Activities

1. Obtain permission to conduct an interview of a school-age child who was recently hospitalized. Some areas to explore in the interview might include:
A. Reason for admission
B. What parts of admission child enjoyed
C. What was frightening
D. What would have made admission a better experience
E. Which staff members child liked or disliked and why

Ask the child to draw a picture about the hospital, and consider how the key features of the drawing reflect the hospitalization experience of a child at this developmental stage.

2. Contact your local school system and investigate their policies regarding the education of hospitalized or homebound children. Some issues to discuss might include eligibility requirements for out-of-school tutoring, educational techniques used in the hospital or home, and strategies used to include the child in classroom activities.

3. Outline an age-appropriate plan of care for a 5-year-old child with a fractured tibia who is undergoing open reduction. Be sure to include both psychosocial and physical interventions.

4. Interview a home health nurse who provides care to pediatric patients. Some areas to explore include how the needs of the family and child are met, what types of equipment are used in the home, what support services are available, and how the services are financed.

ANSWERS WITH RATIONALES

Review of Concepts

MATCHING

1.
1. A, B	2. B, C	3. B
4. B, C	5. A	6. C

SHORT ESSAY

1. The child needs reminders of parents and home. Encourage the family to bring in pictures of the family, pets, and close friends. Place some objects that belong to the parents at the bedside — a music box, a pillow, a cloth scented with the mother's favorite perfume or the father's cologne. An audiotape that contains messages from the family can also help the child to tolerate the separation better. Older children might be allowed to call their parents as often as needed. School-age children also enjoy visits and messages from classmates. Displaying cards and messages on the walls for all to see encourages conversation about family and friends and serves as a reminder of their support.

2. Children benefit greatly from being allowed to experience some of the events that will occur during a future hospital stay. Younger children often benefit from guided tours of the hospital. They can be allowed to try on clothes like those worn by staff members and handle equipment, such as stethoscopes and needleless syringes. In this way, the clothing and equipment will not seem as strange or frightening. Before admission, the child can be shown films or given books or coloring books about the hospital. Simple explanations of procedures can be given, with a doll or teddy bear used as a prop (e.g., if the child will have a cast, a toy/mock cast can be placed on the child's doll or bear). Throughout the preparation activities, emphasize to the child that he or she will be returning home when better.

3. The nurse needs to assess the impact that the hospitalization of one member will have on the entire family. Some areas to explore are:
   A. *Family roles* — How will each member's role be affected? For example, who will assume the normal responsibilities of the parent who is staying at the bedside?
   B. *Knowledge of the child's condition*, treatment, and need for posthospitalization care.
   C. *Support systems* — What supports are available? For example, insurance, family and friends to help at home.
   D. *Siblings* — Are they well informed about the child's illness and expected outcomes? Do they know that they are not the cause of the admission? Are they able to visit? Are their school teachers aware of this major stressor in the family? If the prognosis is poor for the hospitalized child, are the siblings involved in therapy to deal with the stress?

4. A. *Child life programs* — A specialist plans activities to provide age-appropriate playtime that focuses on the psychosocial needs of children.
   B. *Rooming in* — Parents stay at the child's bedside and provide or assist with care.
   C. *Therapeutic play* — Play is the vehicle through which the child can work through fears or concerns.
   D. *Therapeutic recreation* — Adolescent recreation program that focuses on decreasing stress and increasing independence and control.

5. Preschoolers can work through many fears and be introduced to new concepts using dramatic play. Some interventions that would be appropriate are:
   A. Practicing deep breathing and coughing
   B. Putting bandage or cast on doll
   C. Taping intravenous line on doll
   D. Giving "injection" (using a syringe without needle) to doll

Critical Thinking: Application/Analysis

MULTIPLE CHOICE

1. A. Logical thought is not well developed in preschoolers, and two unrelated events may appear to have a cause-and-effect relationship. In this example, the child believes that the pain in his stomach is the result of not sharing his candy.

2. C. Protest is a healthy response by the infant or young child who is separated from loved ones. It reflects the development of a meaningful close relationship with parents. This response can be minimized if the parents can stay with and provide care for the hospitalized child.

3. D. The peer group is a major influence in the life of an adolescent, and separation from peers is very stressful. Peer visitation helps to decrease the stress.

4. A. Siblings are most stressed by the unknown. They may fantasize about the hospitalized child's illness and appearance, and they may fear that he or she will die. Younger siblings may assume guilt for the hospitalization through magical thinking, linking the admission to some action on their part. Visitation allows the siblings to see what is really happening and verify the hospitalized child's condition.

5. D. Timing of teaching is important. When a parent is worried about the child's illness, the teaching will not be as effective. Nurses need to continually assess the parent's knowledge and reteach the information as often as needed.

6. A. Knowledge of the child's developmental levels directs the nurse to teaching strategies that are most effective for that stage of development (e.g., school-age children need to be able to manipulate objects in order to learn about them).

7. B. Repetition of familiar stories promotes a sense of stability in the unfamiliar hospital environment. The other choices are appropriate for older children.

8. C. Peers are important at this age and hospitalized teens derive the most comfort from the presence of their friends. Activities such as a movie help the hospitalized teen feel normal.

9. B. Children of this age associate painful procedures with the place where they were performed. The child will experience less stress when his or her bed is maintained as a safe and pain-free place.

10. B. Many factors that have an impact on discharge teaching are known at the time of admission. For example, if the child has a fractured leg and will be undergoing surgery, teaching will be needed about cast care, neurologic checks, signs of infection, and mobility needs. This information can be taught and reinforced during the hospital stay. Other information (e.g., medications to be administered after discharge) may not be known until close to the time of discharge.

11. A. The Gellert Index is used to assess a child's knowledge of the human body's content and function.

CASE STUDIES

1. A 9-year-old child is old enough to understand the reason for the skeletal traction and should be given a thorough explanation. Pictures of an inserted pin and drawings of the type of traction to be used will aid understanding. Ideally education should begin the day before the procedure, but at minimum several hours before it is begun, to allow the child time to assimilate the information. During the procedure, encourage the child to sit as still as possible, but be ready to restrain the child, if necessary. Continually tell the child what is happening. Encourage stress-reduction exercises such as deep breathing and counting. Allow the child to yell if desired, and praise all cooperative efforts.

2. Much of this 4-year-old child's fear directly relates to the pain and discomfort she is experiencing. Before any therapeutic play techniques can be effective, appropriate measures are needed to control her pain. Preschoolers fear bodily harm, and the open

wound confirms this child's fears that harm will come to her. One technique to help her deal with her fears is to have her draw on a paper body outline the changes she is experiencing. Encourage her to draw in intravenous lines and dressing sites in order to identify any fantasies about these areas. Another technique is to provide a doll or stuffed animal with the same "wounds" and intravenous lines. Include the doll or animal whenever you comunicate with the child, since the child may be more willing to have the doll "answer" truthfully about pain and fear. Playing with safe hospital equipment (e.g., syringes without needles) may also decrease the fear associated with injections and other procedures. Other measures designed to reduce stress and release tension include reading stories, coloring, playing with clay modeling compound or puppets, and using a workbench to pound out frustrations.

Nursing Considerations for the Child in the Community

Chapter Overview

Chapter 5 focuses on the care of children in the community setting. Issues discussed include the role of the nurse in health supervision, health promotion, developmental surveillance, family assessment, care of children with chronic conditions, and home health care.

Learning Objectives

After studying this chapter, you should be able to:
- Describe the nurse's role in health supervision and health promotion for children.
- Discuss the health supervision recommendations for children in specific age groups.
- Discuss health promotion in the community for children with chronic illnesses.
- Describe the rationale for developmental screening.
- Discuss the uses of developmental screening tests.
- List factors in the community that can have a negative effect on a child's growth and development.
- Describe methods to assess a family for strengths, resilience, coping skills, and resources.
- Explain the focus of home care nursing for medically fragile children.

Review of Concepts

MATCHING

Match the age groups in list 1 with the appropriate anticipatory guidance and health education activities in list 2. (*Note:* Items may be used more than once.)

1. Therapeutic Play Techniques

LIST 1
A. Infancy (birth–1 year)
B. Early childhood (1–5 years)
C. Middle childhood (5–12 years)
D. Adolescence (12–18 years)

LIST 2
1. ____ Nutritional needs
2. ____ Rapid growth and development
3. ____ Injury prevention
4. ____ Peer influence
5. ____ Toilet training
6. ____ Sexual activity options
7. ____ Sexual development

Short Essay

1. List three advantages of a health program that emphasized health promotion and health protection.

2. Give two examples of health problems that can be identified in a newborn before symptoms are present.

3. List factors in the community that can have a negative impact on a child's growth and development.

Critical Thinking: Application/Analysis

Multiple Choice

Select the best answer.

1. The rationale for doing developmental screening on young children is to:

   A. Determine child's intelligence
   B. Identify developmental delays
   C. Look for mental retardation
   D. Increase child's skills

2. Which of the following topics is appropriate to cover when giving anticipatory guidance to the parent of a 10-month-old?

   A. Growth will slow dramatically in next 2 months
   B. Once teeth come in, infant will not be putting things in mouth
   C. Raw carrot is a health food for this age group
   D. Infant is at risk for injuries because of increasing mobility

3. A nursing role when working with the family of a chronically ill child is to help the family:

   A. Identify their strengths and areas for improvement
   B. Get health insurance that will cover illness

   C. Find alternative placement for ill child
   D. Interview prospective caregivers for child

4. A useful tool for assessing a family's coping ability and functioning is:

   A. Comprehensive health history
   B. Family APGAR Questionnaire
   C. Discussion of previous crises
   D. Family needs assessment

Case Studies

1. You are approached by a mother who is very concerned about her 8-month-old infant's development. The mother explains that her best friend's infant, who is the same age, is doing many more things than her own child. What information would you gather about this infant, and what guidance would you give the mother?

2. Clarissa, who is 6 years old, was recently diagnosed with diabetes mellitus. After a brief hospitalization, she is now ready to return to school. Discuss preparations that will help with the transition back to her first-grade classroom.

Suggested Learning Activities

1. Administer a developmental screening test (e.g., Denver II) to a toddler or preschooler. Evaluate the results and attempt to explain any delays that you found.

2. Visit an elementary school nurse during a normal school day. Describe the activities performed in the school by the nurse that focus on health promotion and disease prevention, as well as illness care.

3. Contact a home health care agency that serves a pediatric population. Discuss with a nurse the strategies used in the community setting to improve patient and family control over chronic illness.

ANSWERS WITH RATIONALES

Review of Concepts

MATCHING
1.

1. A, B, C, D	2. A, D	3. A, B, C, D
4. C, D	5. B	6. D
7. C, D		

SHORT ESSAY

1. A health program that emphasizes health promotion and health protection has the following advantages:
   A. Promotes optimal well-being
   B. Reduces pain and suffering of children and families
   C. Reduces health care costs

2. Two health conditions that can be detected using screening tests before symptoms are apparent are:
   A. *Phenylketonuria (PKU)* — This is an inherited disorder of amino acid metabolism that affects the body's utilization of protein. Once identified, the child is placed on a diet with very low amounts of phenylalanine, thereby avoiding the mental retardation that would result if the condition were not recognized early. (See Chapter 20 for more information.)
   B. *Congenital hypothyroidism* — This is a disorder in which levels of active thyroid hormones are decreased. Once identified, the child is given replacement thyroid hormones to facilitate normal growth and avoid mental retardation.

3. Several factors that can negatively impact the growth and development of a child include poverty, community violence, poor housing, environmental hazards, lack of access to medical services, and such. When two or more of these factors are present, the child's parents may need extra guidance on how to provide a supportive environment for their child.

Critical Thinking: Application/Analysis

MULTIPLE CHOICE

1. B. Developmental screening is performed to review children's motor skills, language, and behavior milestones with the goal of identifying normal age-appropriate achievement of developmental milestones. If a developmental delay is identified, the child can be referred for additional testing and treatment.

2. D. Infancy is a time of very rapid growth and devleopment. Safety issues include considerations related to increasing mobility, as the infant develops the ability to sit, crawl, and walk. The infant can now reach for and pull objects, increasing the risk of injuries such as burns from hot liquids (e.g., cup of coffee or tea) or pulling a heavy object on the head. Another safety issue is choking, as the infant explores everything with the mouth.

3. A. Families of a child with a chronic condition are dealing with multiple stressors on a daily basis. Many families need help to learn new skills, adapt to changes, and gain confidence in their abilities to manage the challenges they face. Nurses can help families identify their strengths and areas for improvement to increase their resilience in dealing with the stresses and challenges that they must face.

4. B. The Family APGAR Questionnaire is an initial screening tool that focuses on the family's adaptation, partnership, growth, affection, and resolve. It provides a picture of the family's ability to cope with the demands of daily life.

1. The best way to reassure this mother is to perform a developmental screening test. Gather information about prenatal and birth history, illnesses, and nutritional history. If the infant was premature, the number of weeks preterm must be subtracted from the current age when development is being assessed. Administer a screening test such as the Revised Prescreening Developmental Questionnaire. This is a parent questionnaire with age group–specific questions that can be used to assess children up to 6 years of age. It is easily administered and explained to the parent. Many parents are not aware that all children follow the same sequence of development (e.g., all infants will roll over before sitting) but vary in the age at which they achieve developmental milestones. The developmental screening can be used to evaluate the child's current developmental level and to compare it to the norms for that age. This is often reassuring to parents.

2. Clarissa's parents need to contact the school administrator and school nurse to develop an Individual School Health Plan. The plan should be developed collaboratively by the parents, child, school nurse, school administrators, and teachers. It should include information about Clarissa's medications and injection schedule, blood glucose testing regimen, and dietary needs at school and in the afternoon when coming home on the bus. Also, it should outline signs and symptoms of problems (e.g., hypoglycemia) so that all staff can recognize problems and seek appropriate care. Parents need to supply copies of educational material about diabetes for school use as well as the necessary equipment and supplies for glucose testing and insulin injection. Clarissa needs to decide if she wants to discuss her diabetes with her class and, if so, her parents and the nurse should work closely with the school nurse in preparing this program.

The Child with a Life-Threatening Illness or Injury

Chapter Overview

Chapter 6 focuses on the care of a child with a life-threatening illness or injury. Areas discussed include children's response to the stressors of hospitalization, parents' and siblings' reactions to the illness or injury, and the response to death by parents, siblings, the dying child, and the hospital staff.

Learning Objectives

After studying this chapter, you should be able to:
- Describe the stressors of hospitalization for children in various developmental stages.
- Discuss nursing measures that will minimize the stressors of hospitalization in children.
- Identify the five stages of parental reaction when a child becomes critically ill or injured.
- Describe the needs of parents during the hospitalization of their critically ill child.
- Describe the reaction of siblings to the illness of a brother or sister.
- Identify nursing strategies for working with siblings of a critically ill child.
- Discuss parents' reactions to the death of their child.
- Discuss siblings' reactions to the death of a brother or sister.
- Describe children's understanding of and reaction to death according to their age group.
- Examine your own responses to death and dying.

Review of Concepts

MATCHING

Match the items in list 1 with the appropriate word or phrase in list 2. (*Note:* Items may be used more than once.)

1. Stressors of Hospitalization by Developmental Stage

LIST 1
A. Infant
B. Toddler
C. Preschool child
D. School-age child
E. Adolescent

List 2

1. ____ Painful, invasive procedures
2. ____ Separation anxiety
3. ____ Stranger anxiety
4. ____ Loss of self-control
5. ____ Loss of control
6. ____ Fear of dark
7. ____ Fear of death
8. ____ Disfigurement
9. ____ Bodily injury
10. ____ Separation from peer group

2. Children's Understanding of Death

List 1

A. Infant
B. Toddler
C. Preschool child
D. School-age child
E. Adolescent

List 2

1. ____ No understanding of death
2. ____ Death is reversible
3. ____ Death is irreversible
4. ____ Death is a punishment
5. ____ Thoughts can cause death
6. ____ Death is universal

Short Essay

1. Toddlers are at high risk for stress during hospitalization. With developmental level in mind, describe the stressors that have a major effect on the emotional health of toddlers hospitalized with an acute illness.

2. Describe nursing actions that would facilitate the building of a trusting relationship between the parents of a critically ill child and the hospital staff.

3. A mother tells you that she wishes to give her critically ill daughter home remedies to help her get better more quickly. The family has used these traditional medicines for generations, and the mother states that they have always helped. How would you respond to this parent?

4. Parents of a critically ill child are often unaware of the needs of their other children during this time of crises. What anticipatory guidance would you give the parents about their other children?

Critical Thinking: Application/Analysis

Multiple Choice

Select the best answer.

1. Following extensive treatment of a severe bone infection in his leg, a hospitalized adolescent is ready to be discharged. The day before discharge, he complains about the appearance of the large incision on his leg. This response reflects:

   A. Denial of severity of condition
   B. Limited understanding of treatment plan
   C. Regression to earlier developmental stage
   D. Normal concern about body image

2. The best strategy to promote a sense of security for a young child in the pediatric intensive care unit (PICU) is to:

   A. Build a "tent" around bed
   B. Encourage open parental visitation
   C. Allow child to have his or her own blanket or toys
   D. Perform painful procedures away from bed

3. The parents of a critically ill child verbally attack the physicians and nurses who are caring for their child. This response is most likely the result of their:

   A. Concern about child's care
   B. Feelings of anger about child's illness
   C. Dissatisfaction with treatment plan
   D. Lack of understanding of child's illness

4. The best strategy to help parents of a critically ill child maintain their own self-esteem and self-control is to:

   A. Discourage constant visitation
   B. Avoid overburdening them with information

C. Allow them to participate in child's care

D. Encourage them not to express their feelings in front of child

5. Siblings of critically ill children should be:

A. Sent to stay with relatives
B. Shielded from crisis in hospital
C. Allowed to visit in PICU, if possible
D. Reassured that ill child will be fine

6. When bringing parents to the PICU to see their child for the first time, the nurse needs to:

A. Prepare them for child's appearance
B. Caution them against touching child
C. Reassure them that child is doing well
D. Advise that they should leave if they become upset

7. A nursing measure to help a dying adolescent cope with impending death is to:

A. Provide teen with as much independence and control as possible
B. Continue to encourage future planning
C. Curtail visiting by peers to protect teen's body image
D. Allow teen to be alone for long periods of time

8. A strategy to decrease anxiety in children who are dying is to:

A. Tell them not to worry
B. Tell them it is not their fault
C. Avoid any mention of impending death
D. Give them opportunities to discuss issues related to death

9. The best strategy to help the grieving family of an infant who has just died in the PICU is:

A. Encourage them to go home and rest
B. Allow them to hold the infant's body
C. Reassure them that they still have other children
D. Begin arrangement for the funeral

10. The parents of a critically injured child ask numerous questions about their child's condition and treatment. A short time later, they ask many of the same questions again. These parents are experiencing the stage of reaction to their child's injury known as:

A. Anger
B. Shock
C. Loss
D. Readjustment

11. "If I'm real good, and wish real hard, will Grandma come back from the cemetary?" These could be the words of a:

A. Toddler
B. Preschooler
C. School-age child
D. Adolescent

CASE STUDIES

1. A 10-year-old girl was hit by a car while riding her bicycle without a helmet. She suffered massive head injuries and is being cared for in the PICU. What reactions would you expect from her parents, beginning with her arrival in the emergency department through the end of her stay in the hospital?

2. The father of two girls, aged 2 and 4 years, has died in an automobile accident. A week after the funeral, the mother expresses concern about her daughters. The 2-year-old keeps asking for her daddy, while the 4-year-old is not sleeping and is convinced she killed her father. How would you explain these responses to the mother?

Suggested Learning Activities

1. Investigate the policies of the PICU in your hospital regarding patients who are under 16 years of age. Do the policies allow open visitation by parents and siblings? Can parents sleep in the same room with their child? Are the parents allowed to participate in their child's care? Are peers allowed to visit? Are there guidelines for therapeutic play?

2. Identify the resources in your community that are available to support families of children in the PICU. Contact one of these organizations (e.g., Ronald McDonald House), and investigate how it is funded, how long a family can stay there, what services and resources are available, and what the cost is to the family. Interview a family that is currently using this facility to determine if their needs are being met.

3. Caring for dying children is very difficult for nurses, and they need support to enable them to provide the care these children need. Examine your personal feelings about death. Have you ever discussed them with anyone? Have you ever had a loved one or a close friend who died? How did you react? How do you think you would respond to caring for a child who is dying?

ANSWERS WITH RATIONALES

Review of Concepts

MATCHING

1.

1. A, B, C, D	2. A, B, C	3. A
4. B, C	5. D, E	6. B, C
7. D, E	8. E	9. B, C, D
10. E		

2.

1. A, B	2. C	3. D, E
4. C	5. C	6. D, E

SHORT ESSAY

1. Toddlers experience separation anxiety and protest vigorously when they are separated from parents. They cling to routines in their lives and become distressed if their known routines are altered. Toddlers are very active. Through intense physical activity, they learn about their environment. Physical activity is also an outlet for anxiety and stress. Thus it is especially threatening to children of this age group to be restricted and confined in a small area. Other common stressors are fear of pain, invasive procedures, and mutilation.

2. Information is the parents' greatest need, and it must be understandable and timely. Parents need to receive frequent and accurate updates on their child's condition. If changes occur, they should be notified immediately, whatever the time of day. Parents also need to be encouraged to assume the child care activities with which they are comfortable. This enables them to work closely with the staff and to recognize the care providers' concern about their child. Whenever possible, staff should be scheduled so that care providers are fairly consistent since parents' trust in care providers is increased when they recognize familiar faces.

3. A key element of family-centered care is honoring the ethnic and cultural traditions of the family. Many families rely on traditional or folk medicine and would be distressed if these remedies were rejected or ignored. In the situation described, the nurse should encourage the mother to bring in the remedies and sit down with the physician to discuss whether they will interact with the medical treatment. If the remedies will not interfere with the treatment plan, they can be given safely by the family. If they are contraindicated, a thorough explanation of the reasons should be provided (e.g., the potential problems of combining the remedies and prescribed drugs). This approach shows the family that their traditions are being considered and respected and that mutual decisions are being made about the child's care.

4. The healthy siblings of an ill child are also in need of support and attention. Often they feel ignored and left out. Depending on their age, many may be fearful that they will become ill or that they caused the illness. Others may respond with jealousy and resentment. Many have nightmares and fears about the ill child's illness or injury. Siblings need information appropriate to their developmental level. They need to be told about their ill sister or brother in language they can understand. If possible, they should visit the ill child. This enables them to understand the reality of the situation. Often their fantasies are far worse than the reality. In addition, the visits often lift the spirits of the ill child. If visits are not possible, encourage them to send notes, drawings, or recordings. Encourage parents to call the siblings at home on a regular basis to allow them to continue to feel connected to each other by sharing their normal daily activities. This gives the siblings a consistent link to the parents as well as reassurance that they are important and loved.

Critical Thinking: Application/Analysis

MULTIPLE CHOICE

1. D. Changes in body image and disfigurement are major stressors for adolescents. This adolescent is less concerned about almost having lost his leg (because it did not happen) than about having a large scar (because it is permanent).

2. B. Having the parents present is the best strategy for giving a young child a sense of security. The child trusts the parents and is reassured by their presence.

3. B. Many parents react with anger to a child's severe injury or illness, and they may take out that anger on the health care providers.

4. C. Parents were responsible for their child before this illness, and they may feel helpless or worthless if they cannot continue to participate in the child's care.

5. C. Children's fantasies are often worse than reality, and a planned visit to the PICU may relieve many of their fears. The siblings need to be prepared so that they will know what to expect and how their brother or sister will look.

6. A. Parents are often still in shock when they first see their child in the PICU. The nurse needs to describe in detail what the parents will see, including the child's physical appearance and the machines that will be attached to the child. The parents will need the physical and emotional support of the nurse during this visit. They will ask many questions that the nurse should be prepared to answer, even if these questions were answered earlier.

7. A. The normal development of adolescence involves establishing one's own identity and independence. Allowing the teen as much independence and control as possible will meet some of these developmental needs.

8. D. Permission to discuss issues about death helps children feel less isolated and alienated from parents. Contrary to common assumptions, allowing children to talk about death does not increase their anxiety about this event.

9. B. Allow the family to spend as much time as they need with the infant's body. It is the time for them to say goodbye to this child. Other actions that may also be helpful are sending home the last clothes worn by the infant, the identification bracelet, a lock of hair (with family permission), and hand and foot prints and pictures of the infant that were taken after death.

10. B. In the stage of shock and disbelief, parents grope for answers and explanations. They are often unable to assimilate the information they receive, so frequent repetition is necessary.

11. B. A preschooler believes that death is temporary and reversible. This example illustrates the child's use of magical thinking to bring the person back from the dead. In magical thinking, the child believes that his or her thoughts can cause things to happen.

CASE STUDIES

1. Parents' reaction to their child's life-threatening injury usually progresses through five stages:
   A. *Shock and disbelief.* In the emergency department, the parents have difficulty believing that this life-threatening injury has happened. They ask questions again and again, and they do not seem to remember the answers. During this stage, the nurse needs to continue to repeat information and provide support.
   B. *Anger and guilt.* In this stage, the parents express anger at the staff and are quick to find fault with their daughter's care. The parents may feel guilty because their daughter was riding without her helmet. They may also be angry with their daughter if they had instructed her to wear the helmet whenever she rode her bicycle. The nurse needs to focus on facilitating communication with the parents, encouraging them to

express their feelings of anger and guilt so that they can try to put these feelings into perspective.

C. *Deprivation and loss.* As parents begin to accept the reality of their daughter's injury, they begin to mourn the loss of their "perfect" child. They have been their daughter's caretaker for the past 10 years, but now their role has changed completely. The nurse needs to encourage the parents to participate in their child's care as much as possible to help them maintain their self-esteem and self-control.

D. *Anticipatory waiting.* Once their child's condition is stabilized, the parents' concern shifts to the future. Although their questions are now future oriented, the prognosis may still be unknown. The parents may become frustrated by their daughter's apparently slow progress toward recovery. The nurse needs to continue therapeutic communication strategies and to empathize with the parents' frustrations. Answering questions truthfully is essential. Parents also need to attend to their own needs and should be encourged to spend some time together away from the hospital.

E. *Readjustment or mourning.* Readjustment is experienced as the child recovers, improves steadily, and prepares for discharge or transfer. However, if the child dies or if recovery is incomplete, the parents begin the cycle of grief. In either case, emotional support is paramount in the care of the parents.

2. The 2-year old child has no understanding of death. She responds to her father's absence by asking when he will return. The 4-year-old child may be experiencing magical thinking, believing that her father died because she did something wrong (see Chapter 2). The mother needs to explain to her children in simple terms that their father had died, that he will not be coming back to live with them, and that nothing they did caused him to die.

PAIN ASSESSMENT AND MANAGEMENT

Chapter Overview

Chapter 7 focuses on the assessment and management of pain in infants and children. Topics covered include cultural influences on pain, pain indicators, pain assessment, and management of pain (pharmacologic and nonpharmacologic interventions).

Learning Objectives

After studying this chapter, you should be able to:
*   Discuss cultural influences on pain in children.
*   Explore the effect of the caregiver's cultural background in caring for children in pain.
*   Describe physiologic responses and consequences of pain.
*   Discuss the types of pain assessment scales.
*   Describe the differences in children's understanding of and response to pain according to developmental stage.
*   Differentiate between the side effects of narcotic and nonnarcotic analgesics.
*   Discuss the use of patient-controlled analgesia (PCA) in children.

*   Describe various nonpharmacologic interventions to control pain in children.
*   Describe how to prepare children for painful procedures.

Review of Concepts

MATCHING

Match the items in list 1 with the appropriate word or phrase in list 2.

1. Therapeutic Play Techniques

LIST 1
A. Behavioral assessment tool
B. Report of pain intensity tool

LIST 2
1. ____ Poker Chip Scale
2. ____ Faces Pain Scale
3. ____ CHEOPS
4. ____ Oucher Scale
5. ____ Numeric Pain Scale
6. ____ Neonatal Infant Pain Scale (NIPS)

2. Analgesics

LIST 1
A. Narcotics
B. Nonsteroidal antiinflammatory drugs (NSAIDs)

LIST 2
1. ____ Chronic pain
2. ____ Respiratory depression
3. ____ Acute pain
4. ____ Gastric upset
5. ____ Mild to moderate pain
6. ____ Patient-controlled analgesia

SHORT ESSAY

1. List potential physiologic consequences of unrelieved pain in children.

2. Manuel, who is 5 years old, has had abdominal surgery to repair a liver laceration that occurred when he was struck by a car. How would you determine whether Manuel is capable of using the PCA that has been ordered for him? How would you teach him to use it?

3. A 6-month-old infant has had abdominal surgery and returns to the pediatric unit with the following vital signs: T—97.8, P—140/min, R—16/min. The infant is crying and restless. Morphine sulfate has been ordered for pain. Would you medicate this infant? Justify your answer.

4. Describe how to prepare a preschool child for the painful procedure of a venipuncture.

5. Describe the benefits of appropriate pain management.

6. List the clinical signs in a child receiving a narcotic that predict the development of respiratory depression.

7. Nurses have an ethical duty to prevent and alleviate suffering. Discuss ways that the nurse can perform this duty.

Critical Thinking: Application/Analysis

MULTIPLE CHOICE

Select the best answer.

1. A young child may not complain of pain because the child:

   A. Is not experiencing pain
   B. Fears painful injection
   C. Feels pain less intensely than an adult would
   D. Has very high pain tolerance

2. Pain assessment in teenagers of Irish or German descent can be difficult because:

   A. They may exaggerate their pain
   B. They have higher pain thresholds
   C. They may not openly express pain
   D. They will insist on total relief of pain

3. A common indicator of pain in toddlers is:

   A. Quivering chin
   B. Description of pain intensity
   C. Disturbed sleep
   D. Changes in vital signs

4. A child who has been complaining of pain falls asleep. This probably means that the child:

   A. Is no longer feeling pain
   B. Does not need medication
   C. Is escaping from pain
   D. Is exhausted from pain

5. A child's response to pain may be intensified by:

   A. Parental presence
   B. Gently rubbing skin over site
   C. Application of heat or cold
   D. Previous experience with pain

6. The ability to use a pain scale depends on the child's understanding of:

   A. Causes of pain
   B. Concepts of more or less and higher or lower
   C. Logic of cause and effect
   D. Methods of pain relief

7. A pain assessment scale that is useful for measuring pain in neonates is:

   A. Faces Pain Scale
   B. NIPS
   C. Oucher Scale
   D. Eland Color Tool

8. A normal response when a 7-year-old child is about to receive an injection for pain is:

   A. "I don't need it now. I'll take it later."
   B. "I really need this shot to feel better."
   C. "Give it to me in my other leg."
   D. "I'll be brave and not cry."

9. A young boy states that he has no pain following an appendectomy. A possible reason for this statement is the child's:

   A. Belief that boys must be brave
   B. Fear of having more surgery
   C. Ability to be distracted
   D. Actual lack of pain

10. Many parents worry about their child receiving narcotic analgesics because they fear:

    A. Addiction to these drugs
    B. Respiratory arrest
    C. Decreased pain tolerance
    D. Low blood pressure

11. NSAIDs are often combined with opioids to:

    A. Buffer action of narcotic
    B. Decrease side effects of narcotic
    C. Treat pain and fever at same time
    D. Increase effectiveness of narcotic

12. A child's dosage of analgesics should be determined by using the child's body weight and:

    A. Equianalgesic tables
    B. Vital signs
    C. Clinical response to medication
    D. Perceived intensity of pain

13. A common side effect of narcotic analgesics is:

    A. Tachypnea
    B. Intensified pain
    C. Constipation
    D. Fever

14. The nurse needs to remember that NSAIDs can:

    A. Cause constipation
    B. Mask fever
    C. Lead to respiratory depression
    D. Produce sedation

15. Which of the following NSAIDs is contraindicated in children with viral illness?

    A. Acetaminophen
    B. Tolmetin
    C. Aspirin
    D. Naproxen

16. The analgesic antagonist used for respiratory depression caused by an opioid drug is:

    A. Numorphan
    B. Oxycodone
    C. Epinephrine
    D. Naloxone

17. When using EMLA cream, a topical anesthetic, it is important to remember to:

    A. Apply only a thin layer to the skin
    B. Wait 45-60 minutes for the area to be anesthetized
    C. Apply where skin surface is most inflamed
    D. Rub the cream into the skin for maximum effect

1. Seven-year-old Jordan has a fractured tibia and has undergone open reduction and internal fixation of the fracture. On postoperative day 1, his leg is in a cast and he is receiving morphine via PCA. However, he is still very uncomfortable and restless. What pharmacologic and nonpharmacologic interventions would you use to improve Jordan's pain control?

2. One tablet of Tylenol #3 is ordered every 4 hours for a 5-year-old child weighing 48 pounds. Tylenol #3 contains codeine (30 mg per tablet) and acetaminophen (325 mg per tablet). The dosage guidelines for children are:

   Codeine: 1 mg/kg/dose
   Acetaminophen: 10–15 mg/kg/dose

   Calculate the appropriate doses for this child, and indicate if this example is an appropriate prescription. (*Hint:* Refer to the *Quick Reference to Pediatric Clinical Skills* for assistance in calculating medication doses.)

3. Dilaudid 0.32 mg is ordered PO for an infant who weighs 7.5 kg. The oral dosage guideline is 0.06 mg/kg every 3–4 hours. Calculate the appropriate dose for this infant and determine if the dose is appropriate.

4. Three-year-old Jessica is scheduled to have a bone scan. She is very frightened and panics when she sees mechanical equipment, stating that the machines "will eat her up." Describe the best way to obtain good results in the test as well as decrease Jessica's anxiety.

Suggested Learning Activities

1. Examine how you personally respond to pain. Is your usual response similar to that of your own family and culture? How would you react to someone who exhibits an entirely different response? Would it be more difficult to assess this person's pain accurately? Make a list of potential problems that you can identify that would make it difficult for you to accurately assess the pain of someone in a different cultural group.

2. Review the PCA policy in your hospital. Are children allowed to have PCA? If so, what is the suggested age range? Are suggestions available about how to teach a child about PCA?

ANSWERS WITH RATIONALES

Review of Concepts

MATCHING

1.

1. B	2. B	3. A
4. B	5. B	6. A

2.

1. B	2. A	3. A
4. B	5. B	6. A

SHORT ESSAY

1. Acute postoperative pain causes the child to take shallow breaths and suppress coughing to avoid pain; this can lead to possible respiratory complications such as atelectasis and pneumonia. Unrelieved pain may delay return of normal gastric and bowel functions. Anorexia associated with pain may delay the healing process.

2. To use PCA, Manuel needs to understand the concepts of more or less, be able to push the button, and understand that he will receive pain medication when he pushes the button. You should begin by asking Manuel and his parents what words he uses to describe his pain. These words should be used during teaching so that Manuel understands what you mean. Be sure to use only words and concepts that the child can understand. Actual teaching might include the following explanation: "Manuel, when your tummy hurts, you can feel better by pushing the button on the end of this cord. There is special medicine inside this tube. When you press the button, some of the medicine goes into your arm and then to your tummy to help you feel better. If you tummy starts to hurt again, just push the button again."

3. This infant is experiencing respiratory depression, as evidenced by a respiratory rate of 16 breaths per minute. Giving the morphine could cause respiratory arrest. Instead, the infant's vital signs need to be monitored closely and nonpharmacologic measurer used to decrease pain until the respiratory rate increases.

4. A preschooler is able to understand concrete terms. It is necessary to describe what the child will experience in language that he or she understands. A sample explanation might be: "I need to put a small plastic tube into the skin of your arm just like this one. (Show the child a venipuncture catheter.) When I put it in your skin, it will hurt like a prick, but I will put some special medicine on your skin so that you will hardly feel the prick. You can help even more by taking deep breaths and blowing them out of your mouth or telling your mom a special story as I do this. We will help you to stay very still so that it will not hurt too much. If you get scared, it's OK to squeeze your mother's hand very tight and yell "Ouch" really loud. The important thing is to be very still so that we can be done fast. When the tube is under your skin, I will put tape on to keep it there for a while to help you feel better. When you are better, it will be taken out."

5. Appropriate pain management may have the following benefits:
   A. *Earlier mobilization*—with decreased pain, the child is more willing and able to get out of bed and walk, which speeds recovery time.
   B. *Shortened hospital stays*—decreased pain will decrease the complications associated with unrelieved pain
   C. *Reduced costs*—with fewer complications, the cost of the hospitalization is decreased.

6. The clinical signs that predict the development of respiratory depression include sleepiness, small pupils, and shallow breathing. Children who are at higher risk are those with an altered level of consciousness, an unstable circulatory status, and history of apnea, or a known airway problem.

7. The pediatric nurse fulfills the ethical duty of preventing and alleviating suffering by being a patient advocate for the children in the following ways:
   A. Calculating all doses against standard guidelines to determine appropriateness of the dosage. If a dose is too high or low, the physician is consulted to change the dosage.
   B. Evaluating the response to a drug by using pain assessment scales. The child who is having acute pain for several days may be developing a tolerance to the prescribed drug, requiring higher levels of the drug to produce the same effect. The nurse must verify the doses given and the level of relief obtained. If the relief is ineffective, this information is given to the physician and a dosage change is requested.
   C. Using nonpharmacologic interventions to assist in pain control—e.g., parental involvement, distraction, cutaneous stimulation, electroanalgesia, relation techniques, hypnosis, imagery, and application of heat and cold.

Critical Thinking: Application/Analysis

MULTIPLE CHOICE

1. B. Children as young as 6 months of age can demonstrate anticipatory fear of pain. To the child, the fear of getting an injection is more painful than the actual pain experienced.

2. C. Some cultures are very expressive about pain, whereas others are very restrained. Knowledge of these cultural differences in response to pain will enable the nurse to better assess the child's true level of pain.

3. C. Toddlers experiencing pain will demonstrate disturbed sleep. They are not able to describe a specific type of pain or the intensity of pain that they are experiencing.

4. D. Unrelieved pain may cause a child to fall asleep in exhaustion. The nurse should evaluate the sleeping child to see if pain interrupts the sleep or if the child moans or becomes restless.

5. D. A child over 6 months of age can recall painful experiences. This results in fear and anxiety, which increase the intensity of the pain.

6. B. The child must be able to understand the concepts used to quantify pain (e.g., more or less pain; pain is a 4 on a scale of 1 to 10).

7. B. The NIPS (Neonatal Infant Pain Scale) measures pain and distress in young infants using objective criteria for six behaviors or characteristics (facial expression, cry, breathing patterns, arm movements, leg movements, state of arousal). The other choices use the child's report of pain intensity.

8. A. School-age children will engage in bargaining in order to escape a painful experience, such as an injection.

9. A. In the United States, boys are encouraged to be brave and not cry. A nurse can best approach this child by saying, "Most people have pain after this surgery, and getting medicine to help feel better doesn't mean you aren't being brave. When you have less pain, you get well quicker."

10. A. Many people, including nurses and physicians, fear that addiction will result if children are treated for painful conditions with narcotics. Addiction is a rare complication in both adults and children who receive narcotics for this purpose.

11. D. The combination of NSAIDs and opioids increases the effectiveness of the narcotic, which may decrease the dosage needed for pain relief.

12. C. Body weight is used to calculate a starting dose for children. However, the actual clinical response to the drug is needed to determine whether the dosage is appropriate to give relief.

13. C. Constipation is a frequent side effect, and preventive dietary measures such as increased intake of fiber, fruits, and fluids should be instituted. Stool softeners and laxatives may also be ordered.

14. B. NSAIDs have properties of analgesics and antipyretics. Thus the nurse needs to assess the patient for signs of infection continually. If there is any indication of infection, NSAIDs should be discontinued and the patient's temperature evaluated carefully. Alternate pain relief measures should then be employed.

15. C. Aspirin is not given to children because of the risk of Reye syndrome, a metabolic encephalopathy that usually develops after a mild viral illness. It has also been associated with aspirin use at the time of the illness. (See p. 778 for a discussion of Reye syndrome.)

16. D. Naloxone is the narcotic antagonist that is used to reverse the effects of opioid overdose. Caution should be taken to give a dose that will reverse the complication without totally reversing the pain control effects of the narcotic.

17. B. EMLA cream is a topical anesthetic that requires time to be effective. It is applied in a thick layer over intact skin and then covered with a clear adhesive film to maintain the medication in that area. EMLA effectively anesthetizes the dermal layer and is often used for venipuncture and IV insertions.

CASE STUDIES

1. First, have the child identify and locate his pain. Using a pain scale of 1 to 10, ask him to quantify the intensity of the pain. Next, assess the site of the pain. Because the fractured bone is enclosed in a cast, complete neurologic checks are important. (Refer to Chapter 18 for further information.) Have the child explain to you how the PCA works, and ask him to demonstrate how to use it. After he receives a dose, have him quantify the pain again. An appropriate nonpharmacologic intervention would be to apply cold to the cast over the operative site to decrease edema and slow the transmission of pain impulses. Other measures could include having a parent remain at the bedside, distraction (e.g., video), relaxation techniques, and imagery. Continually reassess the child's pain level on the scale. Many children have had minimal experience with pain and expect all pain to be relieved, so it is also important to assess the child's expectations. If pain relief continues to be inadequate and neurologic checks remain normal, notify the physician to reevaluate the child's analgesic needs. The child who continues to have severe pain with no relief is at risk for other complications.

2. The first step is to convert the child's weight to kilograms:

$$48 \text{ lb} \div 2.2 \text{ lb/kg} = 22 \text{ kg}$$

Next, multiply the drug guidelines by the child's weight:

Codeine: $1 \text{ mg/kg} \times 22 \text{ kg} = 22\text{-mg dose}$

Acetaminophen:
$10 \text{ mg/kg} \times 22 \text{ kg} = 220 \text{ mg (low dose)}$
$15 \text{ mg/kg} \times 22 \text{ kg} = 330 \text{ mg (high dose)}$

The acetaminophen dose of 325 mg is appropriate because it falls within the recommended range. However, the child will receive 30 mg of codeine, significantly more than the recomended 22 mg. Therefore, the order of one tablet of Tylenol #3 is not appropriate since the codeine dose is too high. The physician should be contacted regarding a change in the order.

3. The infant's weight is given in kilograms so it is unnecessary to convert from pounds to kilograms:

Dilaudid guideline $= 0.06 \text{ mg/kg}$

Multiply the drug guideline by the infant's weight:

$$0.06 \text{ mg/kg} \times 7.5 \text{ kg} = 0.45 \text{ mg/dose}$$

The appropriate dose is 0.45 mg for this infant and the ordered dose is 0.32 mg, which is not appropriate. The dose is too low. The physician should be contacted regarding a change in the order.

4. Jessica is a candidate for conscious sedation. A bone scan is very frightening to young children. The test is useless if the child does not hold still. Using conscious sedation allows the child to be totally relaxed, be less anxious, and often have no memory of the procedure. Conscious sedation is a light sedation in which all airway reflexes remain intact and the child is easily aroused with verbal or gentle physical stimulation. Many precautions are put in place (frequent vital signs monitoring and advanced life support) should the sedation progress to deep sedation.

8

ALTERATIONS IN FLUID, ELECTROLYTE, AND ACID–BASE BALANCE

Chapter Overview

Chapter 8 focuses on alterations in fluid, electrolyte, and acid–base balance and their implications for pediatric patients. Areas discussed include normal fluid and electrolyte homeostasis and imbalances of sodium, potassium, calcium, and magnesium. A review of the normal regulation of acid–base balance includes the action of buffers and the role of the lungs and the kidneys. Four acid–base imbalances—respiratory acidosis and alkalosis and metabolic acidosis and alkalosis—are described in detail, along with arterial blood gas (ABG) changes indicative of these imbalances.

Learning Objectives

After studying this chapter, you should be able to:
- Describe actions that place infants and children at risk for fluid and electrolyte imbalances.
- Describe the clinical assessment of fluid imbalances in children.
- Identify manifestations and treatment of clinical dehydration.
- Identify manifestations and treatment of edema.
- Describe the clinical assessment of electrolyte imbalances in children.
- Discuss the medical and nursing management of children with electrolyte imbalances.
- Identify foods and substances that are high in potassium, calcium, and magnesium.
- Discuss the normal mechanisms for maintaining acid–base balance in the body.
- Describe the role of the lungs and kidneys in acid–base balance.
- Compare and contrast the four types of acid–base imbalances.
- Interpret ABG results in a pediatric patient.
- Outline potential causes of each type of imbalance.
- Describe clinical manifestations and medical and nursing management of each imbalance.

Review of Concepts

COMPLETION

Indicate the concentration (high or low) of the following components in the fluid compartments listed.

Components	— Extracellular — Fluid Vascular	Interstitial	Intracellular Fluid
Na+			
K+			
Ca++			
Mg++			
*Pi			
Cl-			
Proteins			

*Pi = Inorganic phosphorous

MATCHING

Match the items in list 1 with the appropriate word or phrase in list 2. (*Note:* Items may be used more than once.)

1. Manifestations of Extracellular Fluid Imbalance

LIST 1
A. Volume excess
B. Volume deficit

LIST 2
1. ____ Sacral edema
2. ____ Weight loss
3. ____ Syncope
4. ____ Thready pulse
5. ____ Crackles in lungs
6. ____ Orthopnea
7. ____ Bounding pulse
8. ____ Decreased skin turgor

2. Manifestations of Clinical Dehydration

LIST 1
A. Mild—up to 5%
B. Moderate—5% to 9%
C. Severe—10% or more

LIST 2
1. ____ Thirsty
2. ____ Urine output absent
3. ____ Alert
4. ____ Lethargic
5. ____ Restless
6. ____ Normal skin turgor
7. ____ Rapid pulse
8. ____ Low blood pressure
9. ____ Normal blood pressure
10. ____ Parched mucous membranes

3. Uncompensated Laboratory Values

LIST 1
A. Respiratory acidosis
B. Respiratory alkalosis
C. Metabolic acidosis
D. Metabolic alkalosis

LIST 2
1. ____ HCO_3 is decreased, pH is decreased, and PCO_2 is normal
2. ____ HCO_3 is normal, pH is decreased, and PCO_2 is increased
3. ____ HCO_3 is increased, pH is increased, and PCO_2 is normal
4. ____ HCO_3 is normal, pH is increased, and PCO_2 is decreased

4. Compensatory Responses of the Body to Correct Acid-Base Imbalances

LIST 1
A. Respiratory acidosis
B. Respiratory alkalosis
C. Metabolic acidosis
D. Metabolic alkalosis

LIST 2
1. ____ Increased renal excretion of acid
2. ____ Decreased respiratory rate and depth
3. ____ Decreased renal excretion of acid
4. ____ Increased respiratory rate and depth

1. Describe techniques for accurately measuring an infant's output.

2. List eight manifestations of clinical dehydration in infants and children.

3. List several nursing measures that would be appropriate in caring for a child whose skin is edematous.

4. Explain the importance of maintaining a normal blood pH.

5. Describe how respiratory acidosis occurs and how the body attempts to correct this imbalance.

6. Describe how respiratory alkalosis occurs and how the body attempts to correct this imbalance.

7. Describe how metabolic acidosis occurs and how the body attempts to correct this imbalance.

8. Describe how metabolic alkalosis occurs and how the body attempts to correct this imbalance.

9. Explain how lactic acid is excreted by the body.

Critical Thinking: Application/Analysis

MULTIPLE CHOICE

Select the best answer.

1. Neonates are at higher risk than older children for loss of fluid in the urine because:

   A. They are unable to drink enough to offset urinary losses
   B. They have limited ability to concentrate urine
   C. Their kidneys excrete more potassium
   D. Urinary output increases with fluid intake

2. The most accurate assessment of fluid volume imbalance in a child is determined by:

   A. Daily weighing
   B. Measurement of intake and output
   C. Assessment of skin turgor
   D. Evaluation of areas of edema

3. A potential cause of extracellular fluid volume excess is use of:

   A. Diuretics
   B. Oral rehydration solutions
   C. Nasogastric suction
   D. Intravenous normal saline

4. A safety measure that should be implemented when administering intravenous fluids that contain sodium is:

   A. Use of volume-control device
   B. Giving less fluid than minimum daily allowance
   C. Monitoring serum sodium levels daily
   D. Weighing child daily

5. Extracellular fluid volume deficit can occur when children:

   A. Sweat during strenuous exercise
   B. Have diarrhea and vomiting
   C. Are placed on low-sodium diet
   D. Drink less water than usual

6. Parents should be cautioned to avoid using diet beverages as oral rehydration solutions because:

   A. Sugar is needed for absorption of sodium
   B. Calories are needed for energy
   C. Artificial sweeteners are not safe for children
   D. Diet beverages do not supply enough sodium

7. A bedridden child should be assessed for edema by palpating the:

   A. Abdomen
   B. Fingers
   C. Ankles
   D. Sacrum

8. Giving an infant formula that is mixed with too little water can cause:

A. Weight gain
B. Overhydration
C. Hyponatremia
D. Hypernatremia

9. A simple test to monitor hydration levels in children is:

   A. Urine specific gravity
   B. Hematocrit and hemoglobin
   C. Urine pH
   D. Serum pH

10. When a child is admitted to the hospital with hypernatremia, one possible cause that should be investigated is:

    A. Salt restrictions at meals
    B. Forced fluid intake
    C. Excess fluid restriction
    D. Feeding concentrated juice

11. Hyponatremia can be caused by:

    A. Oral rehydration solutions
    B. Giving water with meals
    C. Tap water enemas
    D. Low-sodium diet

12. A method to measure abdominal edema accurately when monitoring ascites over several days is to:

    A. Measure from base of sternum to symphysis pubis
    B. Mark skin on both sides of abdomen where tape measure is to be placed
    C. Measure at lower edge of rib cage
    D. Place tape measure around abdomen at umbilicus

13. The serum potassium level of a 3-month-old infant is 5.9 mEq/L. The first action a nurse should take is to:

    A. Notify physician immediately
    B. Increase IV rate and monitor urinary output
    C. Determine site from which blood sample was drawn
    D. Assess muscle strength of infant's legs

14. A child is to receive an intravenous infusion of 1L of D_5W with 10 mEq of KCl added. Before beginning this infusion, the nurse must assess:

    A. Hydration status
    B. Urinary output
    C. Serum potassium level
    D. Serum glucose level

15. A child with hyperkalemia should avoid eating which of the following foods?

    A. Strawberries
    B. Apples
    C. Celery
    D. Spinach

16. Children diagnosed with hypercalcemia are at high risk for:

    A. Vitamin D deficiency
    B. Rickets
    C. Tetany
    D. Renal calculi

17. A hypocalcemic child should be encouraged to eat which of the following foods?

    A. Carrots
    B. Lettuce
    C. Legumes
    D. Tomatoes

18. A diet for a child with hypomagnesemia would include:

    A. Oranges
    B. Potatoes
    C. Spinach
    D. Strawberries

19. Assessment of a child with hypomagnesemia would include observing for:

    A. Muscle twitching
    B. Muscle weakness
    C. Slowed reflexes
    D. Lethargy

20. Carbonic acid is excreted from the body in the form of:

    A. Hydrochloric acid
    B. Carbon dioxide and water
    C. Bicarbonate
    D. Carbonic anhydrase

21. Serum P_{CO_2} is an indirect measurement of:

    A. Carbonic acid
    B. Carbonic anhydrase
    C. Bicarbonate
    D. Carbon dioxide and water

22. Which of the following symptoms may be an indication of acidosis in a young child?

    A. Hyperventilation
    B. Lethargy
    C. Bradycardia
    D. Diaphoresis

23. To facilitate renal compensation in a child with respiratory acidosis, encourage:

    A. Voiding every 2 hours
    B. Deep breathing and coughing
    C. Increased fluid intake
    D. Oral intake of bicarbonate

24. Which of the following symptoms may be an indication of respiratory alkalosis in a young child?

    A. Shallow respirations
    B. Tachycardia
    C. Lethargy
    D. Tingling in fingers

25. Respiratory alkalosis is caused by:

    A. Intake of bicarbonate
    B. Hyperventilation
    C. Respiratory depression
    D. General anesthesia

26. Which of the following is contraindicated in a child who has metabolic acidosis?

    A. Codeine
    B. Tylenol
    C. Serial ABG measurements
    D. Cardiac monitoring

27. A child with severe vomiting will develop:

    A. Respiratory acidosis
    B. Metabolic acidosis
    C. Respiratory alkalosis
    D. Metabolic alkalosis

CASE STUDIES

1. The mother of 2-year-old James calls the pediatric clinic to report that her son began having diarrhea 4 hours ago and is now having some vomiting. In response to your questioning, she reports that James continues to be alert and has no signs of dehydration. What actions would you advise James' mother to take?

2. A 3-year-old child is admitted to the hospital with congestive heart failure secondary to congenital heart disease. The child is receiving digoxin and diuretics. Discuss the potential fluid and electrolyte imbalances that this child may experience, and describe how to assess for these imbalances.

3. Theresa has suffered a head injury. She is breathing shallowly and is confused and lethargic. Her ABGs show decreased pH and increased P_{CO_2}. Describe the probable cause of these symptoms and possible treatment measures.

Suggested Learning Activities

1. Examine the policy and procedure manual in your hospital for a policy on administering intravenous potassium. Are there specific guidelines for children receiving potassium? Do these guidelines indicate the importance of an adequate urinary output prior to beginning the infusion? If there is no policy, or if vital directions are missing, how would you go about changing the policy?

2. Interview a pediatrician in your area about guidelines given to parents about care of children with common illnesses. What advice is given for vomiting and diarrhea? Is oral rehydration recommended? Are assessments of the character of the excreta and level of consciousness included? When is the parent advised to notify the physician?

3. Visit the pediatric intensive care unit in your hospital. Discuss the nurse's role in assessment of acid–base balance for children on ventilators. Practice interpreting actual ABG results.

4. Visit a facility that treats adolescents with eating disorders such as bulimia nervosa and anorexia nervosa. Explore the acid–base imbalances usually seen in these disorders. Discuss with the treatment team measures that are instituted to restore acid–base balance. What instruction is given to patients about the danger of acid–base imbalances and measures to prevent these imbalances in the future?

ANSWERS WITH RATIONALES

Review of Concepts

COMPLETION

Components	Extracellular Fluid Vascular	Extracellular Fluid Interstitial	Intracellular Fluid
Na⁺	High	High	Low
K⁺	Low	Low	High
Ca⁺⁺	Low	Low	Low (higher than ECF)
Mg⁺⁺	Low	Low	High
*Pi	Low	Low	High
Cl-	High	High	Low
Proteins	High	Low	High

*Pi = Inorganic phosphorous

MATCHING

1.
1. A	2. B	3. B
4. B	5. A	6. A
7. A	8. B	

2.
1. A, B	2. C	3. A, B
4. B, C	5. A, B	6. A
7. B, C	8. B, C	9. A, B
10. C		

3.
1. C	2. A	3. D
4. B		

4.
1. A	2. D	3. B
4. C		

SHORT ESSAY

1. Urinary and stool output is measured by weighing all dry diapers before use and then reweighing them after use. The difference in grams is equivalent to the volume in milliliters. If an infant is spitting up, weighing the burp cloth before and after use will also determine the volume of emesis. (*Clinical tip:* Writing the dry weight on the diaper or cloth with a pen ensures that the weight will not be forgotten and that it will be available to anyone who cares for the infant.)

2. Manifestations of clinical dehydration include weight loss, rapid pulse, dry mucous membranes, decreased skin turgor, absence of tears, sunken eyeballs, sunken fontanels in infants, and lethargy to comatose level of consciousness.

3. Elevation of a localized area of edema helps decrease swelling (e.g., elevating a swollen scrotum). Skin that is edematous is fragile and prone to disruption either by pressure on the area or by friction. Frequent position changes, careful turning to prevent friction, and frequent cleansing and patting dry (rather than rubbing) are appropriate measures. To prevent the child from scratching the skin, it is helpful to cut the nails short or place mittens on the hands.

4. For the enzymes inside cells to function optimally, the pH of the cell must be within the normal range. If the pH inside the cells becomes too high or too low, the speed of chemical reactions becomes inappropriate for proper cell function. In severe cases, this can result in death. All cells in the body produce acids, which are released into the extracellular fluid and must be neutralized or excreted (via the lungs or kidneys) to prevent dangerous accumulation.

5. The lungs are responsible for excreting carbonic acid (H_2CO_3) from the body. Carbon dioxide (CO_2) combines with water (H_2O) in the blood to produce carbonic acid (H_2CO_3). Respiratory acidosis occurs when there is an accumulation of CO_2 in the blood. (See Table 8–18 for a list of factors that interfere with CO_2 excretion.) As the P_{CO_2} increases, the pH of the blood decreases. The body begins to correct this imbalance by trying to increase excretion of CO_2 from the lungs (increased respiratory rate). If the alkalosis persists for several days, the body begins to excrete other acids through the kidneys to return the pH to normal. This process takes several days to become fully effective.

6. Respiratory alkalosis occurs when the lungs excrete too much carbonic acid through hyperventilation. (See Table 8–20 for causes of hyperventilation.) Respiratory alkalosis results in cerebral vasoconstriction and leads to decreased oxygen perfusion of brain tissue. The body attempts to slow the respiratory rate; however, it may be unable to correct the condition that caused the hyperventilation (e.g., hypoxemia, pain, fever). If the alkalosis persists for several days, the kidneys will retain more acid and excrete more bicarbonate to correct the pH.

7. Metabolic acidosis occurs when there is an excess of any acid except carbonic acid in the blood. This is caused by either an excess of metabolic acids or a loss of bicarbonate, which normally neutralizes these acids. (See Table 8–23 for causes of metabolic acidosis.) When the pH of the blood begins to decrease, the body begins to compensate by increasing the rate and depth of breathing, causing more carbonic acid to be excreted and the pH to rise.

8. Metabolic alkalosis occurs when there are too few metabolic acids. This is caused by a gain of bicarbonate or by a loss of metabolic acids. (See Table 8–26 for causes of metabolic alkalosis.) The body responds to this increased pH in the blood by decreasing the excretion of carbonic acid from the lungs through hypoventilation. Retention of carbonic acid causes the pH to decrease. However, this compensation cannot continue for an extended time because the elevated P_{CO_2} level is not compatible with life, and the need for oxygen will cause the respiratory rate to increase again.

9. Lactic acid is a metabolic acid produced by the muscles. It is released into the extracellular fluid and must be neutralized or excreted to prevent a dangerous accumulation. This acid is neutralized by the bicarbonate buffer system and excreted by the kidneys.

Critical Thinking: Application/Analysis

MULTIPLE CHOICE

1. B. Neonates have a limited ability to concentrate or dilute urine. Thus they are unable to conserve or excrete fluid in response to fluid shifts.

2. A. Rapid change in body weight provides an accurate measurement of fluid volume changes. Every change of 1 gram (g) is equivalent to 1 milliliter (mL) of fluid. Therefore a gain of 425 g of weight overnight means that the child has an increased water volume of 425 mL.

3. D. Extracellular fluid volume excess can be caused by administering an isotonic intravenous fluid that contains sodium. Examples are normal saline, Ringer, and lactated Ringer solutions.

4. A. A volume-control device will prevent a sudden extracellular fluid volume overload.

5. B. Emesis and diarrhea can rapidly deplete the sodium levels in the body, causing a fluid volume deficit.

6. A. Diet beverages do not contain sugar, which is needed if the sodium in the solution is to be effectively absorbed.

7. D. Excess fluid will collect in dependent areas. When a child is bedridden, the sacrum will be edematous; when ambulatory, the ankles and feet will be edematous.

8. D. Improper mixing of the formula introduces a high solute intake without adequate water, which is a cause of hypernatremia.

9. A. Specific gravity tests the concentration of urine against the standard of water. A decrease in the specific gravity indicates that the urine is becoming less concentrated. This test is useful in monitoring children who are being rehydrated.

10. C. Hypernatremia occurs when the body contains excess sodium relative to water. This can happen if an infant is fed improperly prepared formula. However, in one form of child abuse called Munchausen syndrome by proxy, a child may be deliberately deprived of water, causing the child to become ill.

11. C. Tap water enemas introduce excess water to the body, which dilutes the body fluids. Isotonic saline solutions should be used for enemas.

12. B. If indelible marks are drawn on both sides of the abdomen where the tape measure will be placed, serial measurements will be much more accurate. Having only one reference point (e.g., the umbilicus) can be inaccurate because the tape may ride higher or lower on the back.

13. C. Potassium is found in the intracellular fluid. A heel-stick sample contains blood from the pierced capillaries in the tissue. It may also include some intracellular fluid from the tissue cells that were broken when the skin was lanced. Thus the nurse's first action would be to determine the site from which the blood sample was drawn. If the sample was obtained from a heel stick, a second venous sample would then be obtained. If the original sample was venous, the nurse would notify the physician.

14. B. Potassium is excreted in the urine. If the child has little or no urinary output, the potassium will build up rapidly in the bloodstream, causing hyperkalemia, a condition that can be life-threatening.

15. A. Strawberries are rich in potassium and should not be eaten by children with hyperkalemia.

16. D. Measures to prevent renal calculi are necessary in hypercalcemia because the calcium is excreted in the urine. Calculi are more likely to form when the urine is alkaline and concentrated. The calcium will stay in solution in acidic, dilute urine.

17. C. Legumes are a nondairy food rich in calcium. If the child is not able to tolerate milk and dairy products, he or she can be given this calcium-rich food, along with other calcium-enriched products.

18. C. Magnesium is a component of chlorophyll and is contained in dark-green leafy vegetables. Nuts and grains are also good sources of magnesium.

19. A. Hypomagnesemia is characterized by increased neuromuscular excitability.

20. B. Carbonic acid is excreted solely by the lungs, in the form of carbon dioxide and water.

21. A. Carbonic acid is converted in the body to carbon dioxide and water by the enzyme carbonic anhydrase; thus, P_{CO_2} provides an indirect measurement of carbonic acid.

22. B. Lethargy may be an indication of a decreased level of consciousness resulting from acidosis. Other symptoms may include headache, confusion, disorientation, tachycardia, and irregular pulse.

23. C. Increasing fluids, if not contraindicated by the child's condition, will produce a brisk flow of urine, which helps correct the pH imbalance by facilitating excretion of metabolic acids.

24. D. Respiratory alkalosis causes cerebral vasoconstriction, which leads to decreased oxygen perfusion of brain tissue. Digital and circumoral paresthesias (tingling in fingers, toes, and around the mouth) are indications of the neuromuscular irritability caused by the alkalosis.

25. B. Hyperventilation results in the excretion of more carbonic acid than normal from the lungs, which results in alkalemia.

26. A. The body attempts to reverse the acidemia by increasing the excretion of carbonic acid from the lungs. This is accomplished by increasing

the rate and depth of breathing. Narcotic analgesics, such as codeine, are contraindicated because they tend to depress respirations.

27. D. Vomiting removes the normal volume of acid from the stomach, resulting in alkalosis. Because the acids in the stomach are metabolic (i.e., noncarbonic), the resulting imbalance is metabolic alkalosis.

CASE STUDIES

1. The primary goal in James' care is to get an adequate amount of fluid into his body. The best fluid to give him is an oral rehydration solution that is available in pharmacies without prescription. James should be given 1–3 teaspoons every 10–15 minutes. Even if he is still vomiting, some of the fluid will be retained, providing him with water, sodium, and sugar. The sugar allows the sodium to be absorbed, and the sodium is important to prevent dehydration. If a rehydration solution is unavailable, juice diluted to half strength with water may be given in the same manner. Diet soda and undiluted juices should be avoided. If the vomiting does not increase, the rehydration solution volume should be increased slowly. If the volume of emesis continues to increase, or if James becomes restless and his mouth becomes dry, he should be seen by a physician. Intravenous fluids may be required.

2. Congestive heart failure can cause excess aldosterone secretion, which leads to salt and fluid retention by the kidneys. The resulting edema, in turn, increases the workload on the heart. Treatment includes administration of digoxin, which strengthens the ability of the heart to contract, and diuretics, which remove excess fluid and decrease edema. The child is at risk for extracellular fluid volume deficit from the diuretic therapy and for hypokalemia because aldosterone and diuretics increase the urinary excretion of potassium. An additional complication is that hypokalemia potentiates digitalis toxicity.

The following assessments should be performed: serum electrolyte monitoring to detect fluctuations in sodium and potassium levels, cardiac monitoring to detect any arrhythmias, and monitoring muscle strength in the legs. The child must also be monitored for symptoms of digitalis toxicity (anorexia, nausea, vomiting, and bradycardia).

3. Head injuries can cause depression of the respiratory rate, which interferes with the excretion of carbonic acid from the lungs. This results in an accumulation of carbon dioxide in the blood, which decreases the blood pH, resulting in acidemia from respiratory acidosis. Intracellular acidosis develops when the carbon dioxide diffuses across the cell membranes. Acidosis in the brain cells causes central nervous system depression, resulting in symptoms of disorientation, confusion, lethargy, or coma. Theresa is suffering from respiratory acidosis. The character, rate, and depth of her respirations should be assessed frequently. Lung function must be restored. Treatment measures to accomplish this include coughing, deep breathing, suctioning the lungs, or administration of drugs, such as bronchodilators, to assist in improving ventilation.

ALTERATIONS IN IMMUNE FUNCTION

Chapter Overview

Chapter 9 discusses alterations in immune function in children. Pediatric variations in immune response are discussed, followed by specific immunodeficiency disorders, including acquired immunodeficiency syndrome (AIDS). In addition, autoimmune and allergic disorders are discussed.

Learning Objectives

After studying this chapter, you should be able to:
- Explain the normal immune response in children.
- Differentiate between B cell and T cell disorders.
- Describe the clinical manifestations and pathophysiology of immunodeficiency disorders.
- Describe the precautions used in caring for children with immunodeficiency disorders.
- Outline the nursing management of children with immunodeficiency disorders.
- Describe the clinical manifestations and pathophysiology of autoimmune disorders.
- Discuss the nursing management of children with selected autoimmune disorders.
- Outline the nursing mangement of children exhibiting hypersensitivity reactions.

Review of Concepts

MATCHING

Match the items in list 1 with the appropriate word or phrase in list 2. (*Note:* Items may be used more than once.)

1. Congenital Immunodeficiency Disorders

LIST 1
A. B cell disorders
B. T cell disorders
C. Combined disorders

LIST 2
1. _____ SCID
2. _____ Normal B cells
3. _____ DiGeorge syndrome
4. _____ Wiskott-Aldrich syndrome
5. _____ Normal T cells
6. _____ Selective IgA deficiency
7. _____ Normal IgA
8. _____ Lymphopenia
9. _____ Reduced IgA

2. Autoimmune Disorders

LIST 1

A. Systemic lupus erythematosus
B. Juvenile rheumatoid arthritis

LIST 2

1. _____ Fatigue
2. _____ Splenomegaly
3. _____ Pain in joints
4. _____ Lymphadenopathy
5. _____ Treatment with NSAIDs
6. _____ Treatment with steroids
7. _____ Renal involvement
8. _____ Butterfly rash
9. _____ Can disappear in adolescence
10. _____ Can appear in adolescence

SHORT ESSAY

1. Describe how the human immunodeficiency virus (HIV) alters immune functioning.

2. Discuss nursing interventions for a child with juvenile rheumatoid arthritis (JRA) who has the nursing diagnosis of impaired physical mobility related to joint inflammation.

3. Discuss the stresses and support needed by the family of a child who undergoes bone marrow transplantation to treat an immunodeficiency disorder (refer also to Chapter 13).

4. Describe the precautions that need to be taken when a child is allergic to bee stings.

Critical Thinking: Application/Analysis

MULTIPLE CHOICE

Select the best answer.

1. IgE immunoglobulin is an antibody that combats infections caused by:

A. Bacteria
B. Viruses
C. Parasites
D. Fungi

2. Children under 6 years of age frequently become ill because they:

A. Have limited supply of antibodies against common bacteria
B. Are unable to produce antibodies against bacteria
C. Are coming into contact with numerous antigens
D. Cannot yet produce memory cells

3. Symptoms of B cell disorders do not become evident in infants before 3 months of age because:

A. Immune system is immature
B. Maternal antibodies provide protection
C. Exposure to antigens has been minimal
D. Immune function increases gradually during infancy

4. Infection in an immunocompromised infant with respiratory syncytial virus (RSV) can lead to severe respiratory distress and death. A medication that can prevent this is:

A. Amoxicillin
B. Albuterol
C. RhoGam
D. RespiGam

5. The mother of a toddler with AIDS asks if her newborn will be given the standard childhood immunizations. Your response would be:

A. "Only the child with AIDS will have different immunizations."
B. "The baby will not receive any immunizations."
C. "There is no difference in the baby's immunization schedule."
D. "The baby will receive a different polio immunization."

6. Parents of a child with Wiskott-Aldrich syndrome should be referred for genetic counseling because they need information about:

A. Care and treatment of child and other family members
B. Probability of passing defect on to subsequent children
C. Importance of preventing future pregnancies
D. Strategies to minimize transmission of genetic defect

7. Children are at highest risk of becoming infected with the HIV virus from:

A. Transfusion of blood products
B. Maternal transmission
C. Infected siblings
D. Sexual abuse

8. It is important to identify mothers infected with human immunodeficiency virus (HIV) during pregancy in order to:

A. Treat mother through pregnancy, labor, and delivery
B. Watch infant carefully for development of symptoms
C. Encourage mother to have an abortion
D. Deliver infant by cesarean section to prevent blood transmission at delivery

9. Health care workers can place a child with an immunodeficiency disease at risk for serious infection by:

A. Rooming child with another child who is not infectious
B. Exposing child to someone with a cold
C. Giving injection that breaks skin
D. Failing to wear sterile gloves

10. Which of the following findings would lead a clinician to suspect that a child has severe combined immunodeficiency disease (SCID)?

A. Leukocytosis
B. Viral illness before age of 3 months

C. Persistent infections with opportunistic organisms
D. Thrombocytopenia

11. Adolescents who have lupus are advised to:

A. Avoid sunlight and use sunscreen
B. Perform weight-bearing exercise during flare-ups
C. Increase fluid intake to decrease edema
D. Take aspirin only for fever

12. Children with immune disorders, their siblings, and other close contacts should not receive:

A. Hepatitis B vaccine
B. *Haemophilus influenzae* type b vaccine
C. Live oral polio vaccine
D. Pertussis vaccine

13. The best way to prevent the spread of AIDS in the hospital is to:

A. Test all patients for virus
B. Use universal precautions with all patients
C. Use special gloving techniques for patients with AIDS
D. Isolate patients with AIDS

14. Vitamins that are recommended for children with AIDS are:

A. Vitamins C and D
B. Niacin and thiamine
C. Folic acid and vitamin K
D. Vitamins A and E

15. A strategy to combat stiffness in children with juvenile rheumatoid arthritis is to:

A. Encourage bed rest
B. Give warm baths
C. Give diazepam to relax muscles
D. Give acetaminophen for pain

16. Children with juvenile rheumatoid arthritis often take aspirin or ibuprofen to reduce inflammation. As protection from Reye syndrome, they should:

A. Switch to acetaminophen
B. Receive an annual influenza vaccine
C. Take only corticosteroids
D. Avoid children with colds

17. An infant with persistent thrush (Candida) should be evaluated for:

A. Response to antifungal medications
B. Other fungal infection
C. Immunodeficiency disorder
D. Bacterial infection

18. After being informed that their child has AIDS, a family needs to be:

A. Encouraged to express their fears and feelings
B. Left alone to support one another
C. Instructed in their legal rights
D. Given financial aid information

CASE STUDIES

1. Marie, 10 months of age, is admitted to the hospital with diarrhea, a severe diaper rash, oral candidiasis, and acute weight loss. During the workup for failure to thrive, she is diagnosed as having AIDS. The mode of transmission of her infection is unknown. Outline the home care instructions that you would give Marie's parents.

2. Omar is receiving his sixth dose of penicillin for pneumonia when hives, dyspnea, and swelling in his throat develop. What does this reaction indicate, and what action would you take as his nurse?

3. Dora is newly diagnosed as having environmental allergies. This diagnosis was a surprise to her parents because no one in the family has a history of allergies. Dora's symptoms of wheezing and hives were relieved with antihistamines. How would you identify the allergens causing Dora's symptoms, and what instructions would you give Dora's parents regarding her condition?

Suggested Learning Activities

1. Strict laws protect the confidentiality of persons who are diagnosed as having AIDS. These laws were enacted to prevent discrimination against individuals with the disease. Before these legal measures were instituted, children were restricted from school, people were fired from jobs, and others had their insurance policies cancelled in reaction to their diagnosis. Contact your local hospital or a physician's office to investigate how these laws are being implemented.
   A. What information can be placed in the patient's record?
   B. Who has access to the information?
   C. What is the penalty for disclosing information without the patient's written consent?

2. Contact an organization that conducts summer camps for children (e.g., Boy Scouts, Girl Scouts, YMCA, church groups). Determine how the medical officer handles children experiencing allergic reactions.
   A. Is there preparation to handle a severe reaction to an allergen such as a bee sting?
   B. Are there standing orders from a physician to treat minor allergies?
   C. Do children with allergies bring their own medications or bee sting kits?
   D. Are the children allowed to keep the medication with them at all times?
   E. How is the staff of the camp prepared to deal with these emergencies?

3. Visit a grade school in your area. Interview the school nurse about the school's policies regarding attendance by children with AIDS. Questions might include:
   A. Are there written policies governing attendance by children with AIDS?
   B. What education is given to the teachers and staff about universal precautions?
   C. What happens if a child with AIDS bites another child?
   D. Are universal precautions used with every child and adult treated in the nurse's office?

ANSWERS WITH RATIONALES

Review of Concepts

MATCHING

1.

1. C	2. B	3. B
4. C	5. A	6. A
7. B	8. B	9. A

2.

1. A	2. A, B	3. A, B
4. B	5. A, B	6. A, B
7. A	8. A	9. B
10. A		

SHORT ESSAY

1. HIV targets and destroys T cells, which normally provide cellular immunity and protect against most viruses, fungi, and slowly developing bacterial infections (e.g., tuberculosis). As T cell destruction proceeds, cellular immunity is eliminated. Humoral immunity is also affected. Thus, the child is left unprotected against a myriad of infections that are ultimately fatal.

2. Physical therapy is performed to maintain joint function, strengthen muscles, increase tone, maintain body alignment, and prevent permanent deformities such as contractures. Exercises are chosen that do not involve weight bearing but instead exercise joints and muscles with minimal stress on the joints (e.g., swimming). The child should be encouraged to perform the normal activities of daily living. To help with stiffness and pain, the child's regular medication to reduce inflammation should be given at least 30 minutes before expected activity. Another strategy is to use warm compresses on the affected joints to improve movement.

3. Children who require bone marrow transplantation are severely immunodeficient. Having a child this ill is particularly devastating because the prognosis is so poor. Bone marrow transplantation is one way to restore immune function, giving hope to these families. The family needs both emotional and financial support. The procedure can be performed only if there is a histocompatible donor such as a sibling. Then, both the ill child and donor child undergo surgery. Following the infusion of the donated bone marrow, the ill child will continue to be hospitalized for several months until T lymphocyte levels are elevated enough to protect the child from infection. This entire process is very difficult for the family. Another difficulty is that the family is often far away from home and needs housing and travel resources in order to be near the ill child. Also, this period of time is very stressful emotionally because this may be the child's "only hope" to live. Referrals to social services may be appropriate for help with the financial concerns. Other referrals should be made to support groups or other families who are undergoing bone marrow transplantation.

4. Bee stings can cause an anaphylactic reaction in a sensitized individual. The child and family need to know how to respond in the event of a subsequent sting. If the child has severe reactions, an adrenaline injection kit should be carried by the child at all times. All persons involved with the child need to know how to use the kit properly in order to give the injection. The kit needs to be cared for properly (kept out of high temperatures) and replaced when the expiration date is reached. The child should also wear a medical alert bracelet or necklace.

MULTIPLE CHOICE

1. C. IgE immunoglobulins are antibodies that are useful in combating parasitic infections. They also have a part in the allergic response.

2. A. Acquired immunity (humoral and cellular) is not

fully developed until a child is about 6 years of age.

3. B. Infants are born with maternal antibodies in their circulatory systems. This natural immunity lasts only as long as the life of the antibodies, which is about 3 months.

4. D. RespiGam is an intravenous immune globulin (IVIG) that contains antibodies against the respiratory syncytial virus. The immunocompromised infant is unable to produce the antibodies to fight this infection. The antibodies contained in RespiGam were produced in another human and, once infused, will destroy the virus. This is a form of passive immunity whereby the person does not produce the antibodies but receives the antibodies from another source to fight an infection.

5. D. The infant will not receive the live polio virus because of the risk of giving the disease to the immunocompromised child. The killed virus, which poses no threat, is given instead. This risk must also be considered when parents or grandparents who are immunocompromised (e.g., as a result of chemotherapy) live with or frequently visit a child who is receiving immunizations. (Refer to Chaper 10 for further information about immunizations for children with HIV infection.)

6. B. Wiskott-Aldrich syndrome is a congenital X-linked disorder. Thus, the parents need information about how it is inherited and the chances of having another child with the disorder. This will enable them to make knowledgeable decisions about whether to have more children.

7. B. The majority of children acquire HIV from their mother, either before or during delivery. The virus may also be transmitted through breast milk from an HIV-positive mother.

8. A. Studies have shown a significant drop in transmissions of HIV to the infant when the mother is treated with zidovudine (ZDV) during preg-

nancy, labor, and delivery and the infant is given the drug orally after birth. Ninety percent of all children with HIV were infected by maternal transmission of the virus.

9. B. Immunocompromised children can become infected with many different organisms that are common in the environment and that normally would not cause severe illness. Staff members who have a cold should not care for immunocompromised children.

10. C. Children with SCID have an absence of both T cell and B cell immunity. The presence of an opportunistic infection is the cue that leads the clinician to suspect an immunodeficiency disease, because someone with a normal immune system is not susceptible to infection caused by normal flora.

11. A. Lupus often causes skin rashes and photosensitivity. The adolescent needs to protect the skin as much as possible by limiting sun exposure and using a sunscreen of at least sun protection factor (SPF) 15 if he or she must be in the sun. This will decrease the potential for infection, which can result from skin damage.

12. C. Live oral polio vaccine can cause the disease to occur in these children. The siblings and close contacts can also transmit the virus because it is shed in the stool. Children and caregivers can easily transmit the virus due to poor handwashing.

13. B. There is no way to identify all persons who are infected with HIV. Therefore a policy of universal precautions is used for all patients. This policy involves careful handwashing after every patient contact, wearing gloves whenever bodily fluids or excrement are to be handled, proper disposal of secretions, and disinfection of contaminated objects. If there is danger of splash contamination, goggles and gowns must also be worn by all personnel. (See the discussion of "Standard Precautions" in the *Quick Reference to Pediatric Clinical Skills*.)

14. D. Children with AIDS often lack vitamins in their diet. The antioxidants (vitamins A and E, zinc, and selenium) are known to enhance general immune function and should be given at recommended levels.

15. B. Warm soaks and compresses are soothing to the joints and decrease stiffness.

16. B. Reye syndrome often occurs following a viral infection (e.g., influenza or varicella) when the person is taking aspirin. Since these children need the antiinflammatory effects of the aspirin, it is important that the child receive an annual influenza vaccine. The child should also be immunized with the varicella (chickenpox) vaccine.

17. C. Persistent candidiasis can be an early manifestation of several immunodeficiency disorders.

18. A. The diagnosis of AIDS is a tremendous shock to a family, and they need an opportunity to express their fears and feelings. Referrals should be made to social services and support groups at this time.

CASE STUDIES

1. When a child is diagnosed with AIDS, the family is usually in shock. Most children diagnosed in infancy have acquired AIDS from their HIV-positive mothers. Therefore it is essential that Marie's parents be tested and receive appropriate counseling if they are HIV positive. They must be educated about the disease and made aware that there is no evidence that casual contact among family members can spread the infection. Marie's family must be taught how AIDS is transmitted (via blood, urine, stoool, and other body secretions), and how to protect themselves and others. Areas to emphasize include proper handwashing and hygiene, wearing gloves when changing diapers, and proper disposal of stool, urine, and emesis. Gloves also must be worn when treating cuts, scrapes, and other injuries as Marie gets older. When necessary, bleach should be used to disinfect household objects.

   Care of children with AIDS is primarily supportive because there is no cure. Emphasize the need to protect Marie from infection. Minor colds and infections can be deadly to a child with AIDS, so family members who are ill should be kept away from the child. Marie should not receive the live polio virus, nor should any other person in close contact with her, to prevent her from contracting polio. The skin is one of the few defenses against infection available to an immunocompromised child. Appropriate hygiene and meticulous skin care are needed to keep the skin intact.

   Instruct Marie's parents to assess oral mucous membranes often because thrush (*Candida* infection) is common. If infection develops, careful mouth care with lemon-glycerin swabs every 2–4 hours will promote healing. Any sign of infection (e.g., fever, chills, cough, or mild erythema) should be reported to the physician immediately. Fever is the most common sign of infection in immunocompromised children.

   Measures to promote and maintain Marie's health include providing adequate nutrition. Offering small, frequent meals and favorite foods will increase food intake. Careful monitoring of respiratory function is a priority because in many children with AIDS pneumonia develops. Simple blowing games—such as blowing bubbles, cotton balls, or a pinwheel—can help maintain optimal lung expansion.

   Emotional support for the parents and family is essential. Support groups can provide assistance in dealing with their fears. Advise them of the possible adverse reactions to the child's diagnosis.

2. Omar is experiencing an anaphylactic reaction. (Pencillin is an antibiotic that causes a significant number of anaphylactic reactions.) Your first action is to quickly assess Omar's symptoms. If you suspect anaphylaxis, immediately stop the penicillin infusion, call for help, and stay with Omar. Anaphylaxis can progress rapidly to severe respiratory distress, caused by laryngeal edema that obstructs the airway, and can be fatal. (Epinephrine will probably be administered immediately if the symptoms are severe. For a less severe reaction, an antihistamine such as Benadryl may be given and the patient monitored carefully.) Because the allergic response does not stop immediately, careful observation is

necessary for several days. Omar's parents need to understand what has happened and be aware that their son should never receive medications in the penicillin family again. Omar's medical and school records should also note his penicillin allergy.

3. The history is very important because this information can often identify the source of the allergy. Questions to ask Dora's parents include: What symptoms does Dora experience. When did they first appear? How often do they appear? How long do they last? Ask about seasonal variations, or specific timing of symptoms during the day. Explore whether Dora has had exzema, colic, or rashes when new foods were introduced.

Parent teaching includes suggestions on allergy-proofing the home. Many children are allergic to animal dander, and this may cause a crisis in the family with a strong attachment to a family pet. If the family is reluctant to give up their pet, suggest frequent bathing to reduce the dander. Other common allergies are feather pillows, carpets, dust, and cigarette smoke. Parents who smoke should be encouraged to quit. If they are unable or unwilling to quit, suggest smoking only when outdoors and never in the same room as the child. If foods are implicated, teach parents to review food labels carefully to avoid the specific foods or substances.

10

INFECTIOUS AND
COMMUNICABLE DISEASES

Chapter Overview

Chapter 10 focuses on infectious and communicable diseases in children. The process by which a communicable disease is transmitted and the characteristics that make a host susceptible to infection are outlined. The special vulnerability of children is described along with the physiologic response of fever. The use of immunization to prevent disease in children is discussed, including the types of vaccines and recommended vaccination schedule. The side effects, contraindications, and nursing considerations for each vaccine are presented. Reportable side effects of specific vaccines are also listed. The majority of the chapter discusses 19 infectious and communicable diseases in children. Epidemiologic characteristics of each disease are highlighted, along with clinical manifestations, treatment, and nursing management.

Learning Objectives

After studying this chapter, you should be able to:
- Discuss the chain of infection.
- Describe the factors that make children particularly vulnerable to infectious diseases.
- Differentiate between active and passive immunization and give examples of each.
- Outline the recommended schedule of vaccinations for all children.

- Describe the actions and documentation that are mandated when immunizations are given.
- Discuss the side effects, contraindications, and nursing considerations for pediatric immunizations.
- Describe immunization side effects that must be reported.
- Describe the mechanism of body temperature control.
- Describe a positive benefit of fever.
- Discuss the characteristics, clinical manifestations, treatment, and nursing management of selected infectious and communicable diseases in children.

Review of Concepts

TRUE OR FALSE
1. _____ DTaP causes fever and serious side effects
2. _____ All children should get annual flu vaccine
3. _____ Child with low-grade fever can still receive immunizations
4. _____ Two injections can be given in same extremity
5. _____ Premature infants get same immunizations as full-term infants
6. _____ Fever about 102° F (38.8° C) is common reaction to DPT
7. _____ Oral polio vaccine is live virus
8. _____ Written consent from parent or guardian is required to give child any vaccines

MATCHING

Match the items in list 1 with the appropriate word or phrase in list 2. (*Note:* Items may be used more than once.)

1. Types of Precautions Used for Children Hospitalized with Communicable Diseases

LIST 1
A. Strict
B. Airborne
C. Droplet
D. Contact
E. Standard

LIST 2
1. ____ Chickenpox
2. ____ Coxsackie virus
3. ____ Diphtheria
4. ____ *Haemophilus* influenza type B
5. ____ Hepatitis B
6. ____ Mononucleosis
7. ____ Mumps
8. ____ Pertussis
9. ____ Polio
10. ____ Rubella
11. ____ Rubeola
12. ____ Typhoid fever

2. Duration of Maternal Immunity in an Infant

LIST 1
A. Rubeola
B. Rubella
C. Mumps
D. Diphtheria
E. Chickenpox

LIST 2
1. ____ 6–9 months
2. ____ 4–6 months
3. ____ 12–15 months
4. ____ 2–3 months

SHORT ESSAY

1. Describe a characteristic that places young children at risk for contracting an infectious disease.

2. What information must be recorded when an immunization is given?

3. Describe the contraindications and nursing considerations for measles, mumps, and rubella (MMR) vaccines.

4. Describe the rash that occurs in Lyme disease.

5. The fetus of a woman who acquires rubella during the first trimester of pregnancy is at high risk for developing anomalies. List the most common fetal complications.

Critical Thinking: Application/Analysis

MULTIPLE CHOICE

Select the best answer.

1. One degree of temperature elevation causes an increase in oxygen need of:

   A. 1%
   B. 3%
   C. 5%
   D. 7%

2. One benefit of a fever is that it:

   A. Causes child to rest, enabling body to conserve energy
   B. Eradicates organisms that live at lower body temperatures
   C. Causes child to voluntarily increase fluid intake, which helps kidneys eliminate infectious organisms
   D. Protects body from parasites that live at higher temperatures

3. In passive immunization the child:

   A. Is given live organism vaccine
   B. Contracts actual disease
   C. Is given antibodies against disease
   D. Is given killed organism vaccine

4. Current recommendations advocate that this vaccine be given every 10 years:

   A. Hib
   B. Polio
   C. Tetanus
   D. Measles

5. Which of the following vaccines has been associated with adverse neurologic effects?

   A. Pertussis
   B. Diphtheria
   C. Polio
   D. Measles

6. A common side effect of DTP vaccines is:

   A. Fever over 102° F
   B. Redness at site
   C. Joint pain
   D. Rash

7. Trivalent oral polio vaccine is contraindicated if the child:

   A. Has had reaction to pertussis
   B. Has history of seizures
   C. Is immunosuppressed
   D. Is allergic to eggs

8. Which of the following side effects is a reportable event if it follows immunization?

   A. Rash after MMR immunization
   B. Seizure disorder after DTP immunization
   C. Nodule at site of DTP immunization
   D. Altered liver enzymes after HB immunization

9. The most important approach in breaking the chain of infection is:

   A. Treatment with antibiotics
   B. Isolation of ill people
   C. Sterile technique
   D. Proper handwashing

10. An immunocompromised child who is exposed to chickenpox:

    A. Is given varicella-zoster immune globulin
    B. Will seldom contract disease
    C. Has invariably fatal prognosis
    D. Is usually protected by maternal antibodies

11. If untreated, diphtheria can cause death from:

    A. Sepsis
    B. Airway obstruction
    C. Liver failure
    D. Hyperkalemia

12. A dramatic decline in H-flu type B illness over the last decade is attributed to:

    A. Greater resistance to H-flu
    B. Introduction of vaccination for H-flu
    C. Effective education about disease
    D. Development of more effective antibiotics

13. H-flu type B is a signficant health problem for children because it causes:

    A. Flu-like symptoms
    B. Anaphylactic shock
    C. Several severe illnesses
    D. Antibiotic-resistant illness

14. All health care workers should be immunized against:

    A. Hepatitis B
    B. Tuberculosis
    C. H-flu type B
    D. Mumps

15. Treatment for hepatitis B consists of:

    A. Antifungal agents
    B. Antiviral agents

C. Antibiotics
D. Supportive care

16. The bacterium that causes Lyme disease is transmitted by:

A. Tick bite
B. Direct contact
C. Mosquito bite
D. Parasite infestation

17. A common clinical manifestation of mononucleosis in older children and adolescents is:

A. Headache
B. Lymphadenopathy
C. Hepatomegaly
D. Muscle pain

18. The classic symptom in an infant with pertussis is:

A. Black membrane over tonsils
B. Spasmatic cough and stridor
C. Red, raised rash
D. Swelling of lymph nodes

19. Rabies is transmitted in:

A. Stool
B. Blood
C. Respiratory secretions
D. Saliva

20. A child bitten by a rabid raccoon is treated with:

A. Acyclovir
B. Rabies immune globulin
C. Erythromycin
D. Anticonvulsants

21. The characteristic rash of Rocky Mountain spotted fever begins on:

A. Face
B. Back
C. Extremities
D. Chest

22. A pregnant woman who is not immune to rubella should be vaccinated:

A. Immediately
B. After giving birth
C. In second trimester
D. If she decides to have another child

23. A characteristic lesion that occurs in children with rubeola is:

A. Erythematous rash
B. Koplik spots
C. Petechiae
D. Erythema migrans

24. Ineffective treatment of a streptococcal infection can result in:

A. Reye syndrome
B. Toxic shock syndrome
C. Death
D. Pneumonia

25. All health care workers should have documented immunity to:

A. Tetanus
B. Chickenpox
C. Rubeola
D. Hepatitis A

26. Tetanus is transmitted via:

A. Droplet infection
B. Fecal–oral route
C. Contamination of skin wounds
D. Injection into blood

27. An area is flooded and the water supply becomes contaminated with human waste. An outbreak of which of the following diseases might result?

A. Chickenpox
B. Typhoid fever
C. Rubella
D. Tuberculosis

28. When administering acetaminophen to children, an overdose can occur when:

   A. Drops are substituted for elixir dose
   B. Chewable tablets are given instead of elixir
   C. It is given on an empty stomach
   D. It is given every 5 hours

CASE STUDY

1. Maryanne, 18 months of age, was admitted to the hospital with febrile seizures resulting from a sudden high fever. After 3 days the fever dropped and an erythematous, maculopapular rash appeared, starting on the trunk and spreading to the face, neck, and extremeties. Roseola was diagnosed. What information would you give Maryanne's parents about the disease and about her care after discharge?

Suggested Learning Activities

1. Visit a physician's office or clinic that gives immunizations to children. Observe the preparation and administration of the vaccines and the documentation required. Review the materials given to parents before they consent to the administration of various vaccines. Interview the staff to determine what verbal and written instructions are given to parents. Have staff members ever witnessed a severe reaction to an immunization?

ANSWERS WITH RATIONALES

Review of Concepts

TRUE OR FALSE

1. T
2. F (annual flu vaccines are recommended only for children with chronic conditions, e.g., asthma)
3. T
4. T
5. T
6. F (fever less than 102° F (38.8° C) is a common reaction to DPT)
7. T
8. T

MATCHING

1.

1. B, D	2. D	3. C, D
4. C	5. A, E	6. E
7. C	8. C	9. E
10. C	11. B	12. D

2.

1. B	2. D	3. A, C
4. E		

SHORT ESSAY

1. Young children are at risk of contracting an infectious disease because their immune systems are not fully functional and they have not yet developed antibodies to many agents. Therefore they cannot defend against disease as well as older children. Disease transmission is facilitated by the poor hygiene of young children. Children are often grouped with other children in day care centers or babysitting groups so they easily pass infections to each other. Fecal–oral and respiratory routes are the most common sources of infection because they do not wash their hands without supervision. They also put toys and their hands in their mouths and then rub their eyes and nose.

2. The following information must be recorded when giving immunizations:
   A. Date of administration (mo/day/yr)
   B. Vaccine given
   C. Manufacturer
   D. Lot number and expiration date
   E. Site and route of administration
   In addition, any severe reaction to an immunization must be reported to the state health department.

3. A. *Contraindications for MMR* — Allergy to neomycin and eggs; immunosupression; administration of immune serum globulin or blood products in the past 3–11 months; pregnancy.
   B. *Nursing considerations* — Determine whether child is allergic to neomycin or eggs or immunosuppressed; if so, do not give MMR. Instruct adolescents of childbearing age to avoid pregnancy for 3 months after immunizations.

4. Lyme disease is characterized by a slowly expanding red rash, called erythema migrans, at the site of the bite. The rash starts as a flat or raised red area and may progress to partial clearing, develop blisters or scabs at the center, or have a bluish discoloration.

5. Infants with congenital rubella syndrome can be born with:
   A. Cardiac defects
   B. Ophthalmologic disturbances (blindness, cataracts)
   C. Mental and physical retardation
   D. Deafness
   E. Neurologic complications

Critical Thinking: Application/Analysis

MULTIPLE CHOICE

1. D. The oxygen need increases by 7% and the respiratory rate by 4 breaths/min for each degree of temperature elevation. For this reason oxygenation levels of children who are feverish must be monitored closely.

2. B. Many organisms can live only within a narrow temperature range and are killed when body temperature is elevated. For this reason many physicians do not recommend giving antipyretics for moderate fever.

3. C. Passive immunization involves giving a child antibodies produced by another host that will react to a specific antigen to which the child has been exposed. This method of immunization is used when the child needs immediate protection and there is insufficient time for the body to produce its own antibodies (a process that takes several days). For example, when the child is exposed to a virulent antigen such as rabies, by the time the body produced antibodies the child would already have the disease and the antibodies would be unable to fight the mature infection. In this example rabies immune globulin would be given as soon as possible after exposure, followed by doses of rabies vaccine to initiate the active immunization against the disease.

4. C. Tetanus immunization should be given a minimum of every 10 years and more often if a person is injured (particularly for injuries resulting in puncture wounds).

5. A. Pertussis (vaccine) has been linked to adverse side effects; however, a new acellular, highly refined pertussis vaccine now available has less potential for serious side effects.

6. B. DTP side effects include redness, pain, nodules at the injection site, temperature elevation to 101° F, drowsiness, fussiness, and/or anorexia.

7. C. Oral polio vaccine is a live virus that is shed in the stool. If the child is immunocompromised (e.g., has AIDS or is receiving chemotherapy), he or she can develop the disease. If a family member is immunocompromised, that person can be infected by the virus shed in the child's stool. In both situations the child should be given injectable inactivated polio vaccine rather than the oral vaccine.

8. B. A residual seizure disorder that occurs after DTP immunization must be reported to the U.S. Department of Health and Human Services.

9. D. Handwashing before giving care and after all diaper changes is an important measure in controlling and preventing the spread of infection.

10. A. Immunocompromised children are at risk for death if they develop chickenpox. The immunoglobulin is given as soon as possible after exposure.

11. B. In serve cases children with diphtheria may develop a membranous lesion that covers the tonsils and can spread to cover the soft and hard palates and the posterior portion of the pharynx.

12. B. Vaccination against H-flu type B was introduced several years ago, and dramatic declines in illnesses caused by this bacteria have been noted.

13. C. H-flu type B can cause several severe illnesses, including meningitis, epiglottitis, pneumonia, septic arthritis, and cellulitis. If untreated, H-flu type B can result in death.

14. A. Health care workers are at risk for exposure to hepatitis B in the hospital setting.

15. D. There is no cure for hepatitis B; hence the treatment is supportive.

16. A. The tick transmits the spirochete when it draws blood.

17. B. Mononucleosis causes lymphadenopathy and sore throat. Pain from the tonsils and lymph nodes may be significant.

18. B. The cough in pertussis becomes severe and is characteristically spasmodic. The infant can have apneic spells because air cannot enter the lungs during the coughing episode. At the end of the spasm, there is a sudden inspiration, stridor, or "whooping" sound. The coughing may last 1–4 weeks or longer.

19. D. Rabies virus is present in the saliva and cerebrospinal fluid of infected animals. An animal bite injects the saliva directly into the wound. People who are exposed to the saliva, even if not bitten, are usually given rabies immune globulin and rabies vaccine, because the disease is fatal to humans without immunization. Once symptoms begin, there is no effective treatment.

20. B. Rabies is a deadly disease and the human body is unable to quickly produce enough antibodies to destroy the virus, resulting in infection and usually death. Rabies immune globulin contains antibodies that destroy the virus. These antibodies were produced in another host animal. This is a form of passive immunity.

21. C. The rash begins on the extremities, including the palms and soles of the feet, and moves to the trunk.

22. B. To reduce the risk of acquiring rubella at the beginning of a future pregnancy, the woman should receive the vaccine after she gives birth. Caution her to avoid becoming pregnant for at least 3 months after receiving the vaccine.

23. B. Koplik spots appear in the mouth about 2 days before and after onset of rash. They are small, irregular, bluish-white spots on a red background.

24. B. If a streptococcal infection is untreated, toxic shock syndrome can occur as well as acute rheumatic fever, acute glomerulonephritis, bacteremia, and necrotizing fasciitis or myositis. For this reason, it is very important that all sore throats be cultured and treated if strep is diagnosed.

25. C. All health care workers should have documented immunity to rubeola.

26. C. The spores of the tetanus bacillus exist in soil, dust, and animal excretions and are transmitted through wounds in the skin from contact with contaminated soil or implements.

27. B. Typhoid fever is transmitted through ingestion of food or water contaminated with human waste. This disease causes significant morbidity in underdeveloped countries.

28. A. Acetaminophen comes in several commercially prepared strengths and they can be confused. The liquid preparations are (1) drops, which are more concentrated (80 mg/0.8 mL), and (2) elixir (80 mg/2.5 mL) and they can be accidentally interchanged. There are also two strengths of chewable tablets—80 mg and 160 mg per tablet. Many infants and children are poisoned each year when their parents give them the wrong strength of medication. For example, suppose 80 mg was ordered. The parent was told to give a half teaspoon of elixir but has drops at home. If parent gives the drops instead of the elixir, the infant would receive 250 mg instead of 80 mg—*triple* the dose.

CASE STUDY

1. Maryanne's parents will be very concerned because of the sudden high fever, seizures, and rash. They may initially believe that their daughter has measles. First, reassure them that she does not have either rubella or rubeola. Explain that roseola is a self-limiting disease and, although there is no treatment, the prognosis is excellent. It is not possible to provide information on transmission and period of communicability because these aspects of the disease process remain unknown. Explain that the febrile seizures occurred because of the rapid rise in temperature and are not a manifestation of the disease itself (see Chapter 18). Reassure the parents that Maryanne's rash will disappear in a few days.

ALTERATIONS IN RESPIRATORY FUNCTION

Chapter Overview

Chapter 11 focuses on acute and chronic conditions that cause respiratory dysfunction in infants and children. The anatomy and physiology of adult and pediatric respiratory systems are compared, and urgent respiratory threats are discussed. Reactive airway disorders, lower airway disorders, and injuries of the respiratory system are then presented.

Learning Objectives

After studying this chapter, you should be able to:
- Explain the significance of the differences between adult and pediatric respiratory tracts.
- Differentiate between early and late symptoms of respiratory distress.
- Describe the nursing assessments performed on children in respiratory distress.
- Describe the needs of the family of an infant who has died of sudden infant death syndrome (SIDS).
- Differentiate among the types of reactive airway disorders.
- Explain the nursing management of children with acute and chronic respiratory disorders.
- Discuss the medications frequently used to manage acute and chronic respiratory disorders.
- Formulate discharge instructions for children with acute or chronic respiratory disorders.
- Explain the multisystem changes that occur in children with cystic fibrosis.
- Outline anticipatory guidance for parents of children who have unintentional injuries of the respiratory system.

Review of Concepts

COMPLETION

Compare each of the following airway structures in an adult and a young child. Describe the differences noted and explain their significance.

Structure	Pediatric Differences	Significance
Airway		
Nasopharynx		
Nares		
Tongue		
Epiglottis		

Structure	Pediatric Differences	Significance
Larynx and glottis		
Thyroid, cricoid, and tracheal cartilages		
Tonsils and adenoids		

MATCHING

Match the items in list 1 with the appropriate word or phrase in list 2. (*Note:* Items may be used more than once.)

1. Clinical Manifestations of Respiratory Failure

LIST 1
A. Initial sign
B. Early decompensation
C. Severe hypoxia

LIST 2

1. ____ Dyspnea
2. ____ Retractions
3. ____ Tachypnea
4. ____ Confusion
5. ____ Cyanosis
6. ____ Grunting
7. ____ Tachycardia
8. ____ Restlessness
9. ____ Bradycardia

2. Reactive Airway Disorders

LIST 1
A. Laryngotracheobronchitis
B. Epiglottitis
C. Asthma

LIST 2
1. ____ Drooling
2. ____ Stridor
3. ____ Dysphagia
4. ____ Productive cough
5. ____ Viral infection
6. ____ Bacterial infection
7. ____ Expiratory wheezing
8. ____ "Barking" cough
9. ____ Bronchospasm

3. Medications Used to Treat Asthma

LIST 1
A. Albuterol
B. Theophylline
C. Cromolyn sodium
D. Corticosteroids

LIST 2
1. ____ Ineffective when wheezing is present
2. ____ Rapid-acting bronchodilator
3. ____ Effectiveness depends on maintaining optimum serum level
4. ____ Decreases swelling in mucous membranes
5. ____ Taken daily to prevent asthma attack
6. ____ Common side effects are restlessness and vomiting
7. ____ Often given by aerosol during acute attack
8. ____ Side effects include fluid retention and mood alteration

SHORT ESSAY

1. Parents of an infant who has died of SIDS are often not aware of the needs of their other children. Describe the possible reactions that children may experience following the death of a sibling.

2. Describe three signs of respiratory distress that are seen primarily in infants and children.

3. Corticosteroids and bronchodilators are often used together to treat asthma. Describe the rationale behind this practice.

4. Children with cystic fibrosis are at risk for salt depletion in warm weather because of the loss of salt in their sweat. Outline an educational plan that addresses this problem.

Critical Thinking: Application/Analysis

MULTIPLE CHOICE

Select the best answer.

1. New parents ask your advice about preventing SIDS. You would explain that the incidence of SIDS is decreased when the infant:

    A. Sleeps in an infant seat
    B. Is positioned on side or back for sleep
    C. Is positioned on abdomen for sleep
    D. Always sleeps with parents

2. The emergency department nurse can best support the family of an infant who has died of SIDS by:
    A. Discouraging family from agreeing to an autopsy, since it will be inconclusive
    B. Asking family what funeral arrangements they wish to make and initiating the process
    C. Encouraging parents to hold and touch the dead infant and say goodbye
    D. Encouraging parents to have another baby to replace this infant

3. The nurse's first action in responding to a child with tachypnea, grunting, and retractions is to:

    A. Observe for additional symptoms
    B. Apply apnea monitor
    C. Administer oxygen
    D. Place child upright

4. A child is brought to the emergency department with a sore throat, anxiety, refusal to speak, and drooling. A top priority is to:

    A. Avoid placing anything in child's mouth
    B. Have child drink some water
    C. Inspect child's throat for infection
    D. Draw blood for arterial blood gas evaluation

5. A potential complication of laryngotracheobronchitis (LTB) is:

    A. Strep throat
    B. Bacterial pneumonia
    C. Asthma
    D. Airway obstruction

6. Children with croup need to be well hydrated because fluids:

    A. Soothe their throats
    B. Help to liquify secretions
    C. Improve their cough
    D. Prevent dehydration

7. When assessing a child who is having an acute asthma attack, your first priority is to:

    A. Evaluate child's hydration status
    B. Take child's temperature and blood pressure
    C. Auscultate lung bases for air movement
    D. Determine what medication has been given at home

8. A useful tool for identifying when obstruction is beginning to occur in asthma is:

    A. Spirometer
    B. Peak expiratory flow meter
    C. Nebulizer
    D. Metered dose inhaler

9. Which of the following is an appropriate response by the family of a child with asthma?

    A. Maintain temperature of home at 72° F (22.2°C)
    B. Forbid smoking in home
    C. Keep dogs away from child
    D. Keep child indoors during winter

10. A medication used to prevent asthma attacks is:

    A. Cromolyn sodium
    B. Albuterol
    C. Theophylline
    D. Beclomethasone

11. Infants develop bronchopulmonary dysplasia as a result of:

    A. Chronic infections
    B. Positive-pressure ventilation
    C. Meconium aspiration at birth
    D. Chronic low oxygen levels

12. An ominous sign in an infant with bronchiolitis is:

    A. Diminished breath sounds
    B. Wheezing in bronchi
    C. Crackles in lungs
    D. Refusal to drink

13. Which of the following provides a quick method of evaluating oxygenation status in infants?

    A. Respiratory rate
    B. Heart rate
    C. Arterial blood gases
    D. Capillary refill

14. Pancrease (a pancreatic enzyme supplement) is given to a child with cystic fibrosis:

    A. Each time child eats something
    B. When stools become large and foul smelling
    C. Between meals and at bedtime
    D. When child's appetite begins to diminish

15. A child with cystic fibrosis is at risk for deficiency in vitamins:

    A. B_1 and folic acid
    B. B_{12} and niacin
    C. C and B_6
    D. A and D

16. Children with cystic fibrosis are at risk during hot weather or after strenuous exercises because they:

    A. Lose excess salt
    B. Begin to hyperventilate
    C. Catch colds easily
    D. Do not cough as well

17. When a child is diagnosed with cystic fibrosis, the news is often met with disbelief because:

    A. Family is not prepared to handle chronically ill child
    B. Denial is first stage of grieving process
    C. Parents are not aware that they both carry gene for cystic fibrosis
    D. Few parents have heard of this rare disorder

18. Mucolytic agents are often administered to children with cystic fibrosis to:

    A. Stop formation of thick mucus
    B. Increase production of normal mucus
    C. Decrease swelling in bronchioles
    D. Facilitate removal of pulmonary secretions

19. Chest physiotherapy in cystic fibrosis is extremely important because it mobilizes secretions in the pulmonary tree and:

    A. Decreases child's need for bronchodilators
    B. Increases level of carbon dioxide in alveoli
    C. Stimulates child to breathe more deeply
    D. Helps prevent respiratory infections

20. Sesame seeds are an inappropriate snack for a toddler because the seeds are:

    A. Easily aspirated
    B. Poorly digested
    C. Difficult to swallow
    D. High in fat

21. When caring for a child with a chest tube, a nursing priority is to:

    A. Monitor blood pressure and pulse
    B. Assess oximetry levels continuously
    C. Administer oxygen continuously
    D. Monitor breath sounds in both lungs

22. Teaching a 4-year-old child about asthma can be accomplished best by:

A. Carefully explaining the disease process
B. Dramatic play using puppets representing parts of the lung
C. Drawing simplified diagrams of the lungs
D. Reading a story about asthma

CASE STUDIES

1. Michael, 3 weeks old, is rushed to the local hospital when he suddenly stops breathing. Although Michael's mother had a healthy pregnancy, he was born prematurely at 35 weeks' gestation and weighed 5½ pounds when he left the hospital 2 days after birth. Michael's mother had just finished giving him his morning bottle when he suddenly stopped breathing. Quickly she raised Michael's head and brought him to a sitting position. Michael then began to breathe again on his own. At the local emergency department, Michael's mother tells staff that he had just dozed off to sleep when "He turned blue around his lips and seemed to go limp for about 30 seconds." Michael has experienced an episode of apnea of prematurity. What discharge instructions would be appropriate for his family?

2. A child arrives in the emergency department with fever, sore throat, tachycardia, drooling, and tachypnea. What symptom alerts you to the possible diagnosis of epiglottitis? What interventions are appropriate for a child with this diagnosis?

Suggested Learning Activities

1. Two children, ages 5 and 14, are newly diagnosed with asthma. Outline an educational plan for each child, indicating what information should be taught and how you would present this information. Be sure to incorporate developmental considerations for preschool and adolescent children in your plan.

2. Contact an organization in your area that deals with chronic respiratory diseases (e.g., American Lung Association or Cystic Fibrosis Foundation). Determine what services and materials they offer to the public.

3. Perform a complete respiratory assessment on a healthy child (inspection, palpation, percussion, and auscultation). Document your findings.

ANSWERS WITH RATIONALES

Review of Concepts

COMPLETION

Structure	Pediatric Differences	Significance
Airway	Shorter and narrower	Increased airway resistance; easily obstructed
Nasopharynx	Smaller	Infection can cause obstruction of airway
Nares	Smaller	Easily occluded, especially in infants who are obligatory nose breathers
Tongue	Larger	Higher risk for obstruction
Epiglottis	Long and floppy	Swelling can cause obstruction of airway
Larynx and glottis	Higher in neck	Increased risk of aspiration
Thyroid, cricoid, and tracheal cartilages	Immature	Airway can easily collapse when neck is flexed or hyperextended
Tonsils and adenoids	Larger in early childhood	Increased airway resistance; easily obstructed

MATCHING

1.
1. C	2. B	3. A
4. B	5. C	6. B
7. A	8. A	9. C

2.
1. B	2. A	3. B
4. C	5. A	6. B
7. C	8. A	9. C

3.
1. C	2. A	3. B
4. D	5. C	6. B
7. A	8. D	

SHORT ESSAY

1. Siblings may fear that they will also die from SIDS and may resist going to sleep at night. Preschoolers may have secretly wished that the infant would die or leave their home. They may believe that these thoughts actually caused the death. (See Chapter 2 regarding magical thinking.) Siblings need to be included in any counseling or support groups after the infant's death.

2. A. *Nasal flaring:* To get more air into the lungs, the infant will open the nares as wide as possible during inspiration.
   B. *Grunting:* To keep air in the lungs a little longer, the infant or child will partially close the glottis during expiration, increasing the pressure in the chest. The partially closed glottis forces the air through the vocal cords, giving a vocal quality to the grunting sound made on expiration.
   C. *Retractions:* Drawing in of the skin of the neck and/or chest on inhalation. This skin movement may be seen between the ribs and above or below the rib cage.

3. During an asthma attack, the airway becomes severely narrowed as the mucous membrane lining the bronchi swells and produces large amounts of mucus that plugs the narrowed airway. When this swelling occurs, the smooth muscle in the outer layer of the bronchi goes into spasm, further narrowing the airway. Corticosteroids are antiinflammatory agents that decrease swelling in inflamed tissues in the inner lumen of the airway. Bronchodilators relax the smooth muscle that surrounds the bronchi and bronchioles in the airway. Therefore both work together, but in different ways, to increase the size of the airway lumen.

4. Salt and fluid intake need to be increased during warm weather. Foods such as salted snacks and carbonated beverages are encouraged. As perspiration increases, extra fluids and salt are needed. The child and parents must know how to recognize symptoms of salt depletion (fatigue, weakness, abdominal pain, and vomiting) and should contact the child's physician if these symptoms appear. They also need to keep this problem in mind when planning vacations (e.g., they should avoid hot climates).

Critical Thinking: Application/Analysis

MULTIPLE CHOICE

1. B. Research has shown a relationship between SIDS and sleeping on the abdomen.

2. C. Viewing the infant allows the parents to say goodbye. Before bringing the infant to parents, take footprints and handprints, cut a small lock of hair, and give them to the parents in an envelope. Carefully wash the infant and dress in clean clothing and blanket. Prepare the family for the infant's physical appearance and stay with them, if they wish, to answer any questions about the infant's appearance.

3. D. The upright position assists diaphragmatic breathing and promotes airway patency.

4. A. Manipulation of the mouth or throat can cause immediate laryngospasm and complete obstruction of the airway.

5. D. Airway obstruction is a potential complication of LTB when the upper airway is swollen. The child must be observed continuously for inability to swallow, absence of voice sounds, increasing respiratory distress, and drooling. Children are at risk because their airways are small and narrow and easily obstructed by edema and secretions.

6. B. Fluid needs must be met in a child with croup to liquify secretions in the airway and help prevent obstruction. Liquids also provide calories for energy.

7. C. Oxygenation of the blood requires constant exchange of air in the alveoli. In an asthma attack fresh air is prevented from reaching the alveoli because the airways are plugged with mucus.

8. B. The peak expiratory flow meter measures the child's ability to push air forcefully out of the lungs. The readings are compared to the child's normal baseline and effectiveness of treatment can be confirmed by improved readings.

9. B. Passive smoke inhalation has been linked to the increased severity of asthma in children of parents who smoke.

10. A. Cromolyn sodium is a medication that is only taken prophylactically to prevent an asthma attack. It must be taken regularly but if wheezing does begin, it must be immediately discontinued and bronchodilators started.

11. B. Bronchopulmonary dysplasia is a condition that results from the treatment given to infants with severe respiratory problems. Treatment measures that contribute to this condition are high oxygen concentrations, intubation, and long-term positive-pressure ventilation.

12. A. Diminished breath sounds indicate obstructed airflow through the bronchioles. Trapping of air in the alveoli prevents normal gas exchange, leading to respiratory failure.

13. D. Delayed capillary refill is a sign of respiratory distress. It is easily assessed by stroking an infant's foot or pinching a finger or toenail in older infants and children. (See Chapter 3.)

14. A. In cystic fibrosis the pancreatic ducts become plugged with thick mucus so that the normal pancreatic enzymes are not secreted into the duodenum. For digestion to occur, supplemental enzymes must be ingested at the same time as food.

15. D. Vitamins A and D are fat soluble. A child with cystic fibrosis may have difficulty digesting fats because of the absence of pancreatic enzymes. As a result, the fat-soluble vitamins are excreted in the stool with the undigested fats.

16. A. Children with cystic fibrosis lose more than normal amounts of salt in their sweat. They are at risk for severe salt depletion during hot weather or after exercise. They need to add salt to their diet or eat a salty snack and drink fluids as prevention.

17. C. Cystic fibrosis is an inherited autosomal recessive disorder, which means that both parents must carry the gene in order for a child to have the disease. In past generations most children with cystic fibrosis died very young, often without ever being diagnosed. Families are often unaware that they are carriers of this disorder.

18. D. Mucolytic agents help to thin and liquify tenacious mucus in the bronchioles, making it easier to clear the bronchioles and maintain airway patency.

19. D. Chest physiotherapy helps to remove the thick mucus in the airways. This mucus is an excellent medium for bacterial growth.

20. A. Toddlers have very few teeth, and they are unable to chew the seeds properly before swallowing. The small seeds are easily inhaled by the young child. In addition, diagnosis may be delayed because of the inability to visualize the seeds on x-ray.

21. D. A chest tube is inserted to reinflate a collapsed or partially collapsed lung. The presence of lung sounds in both lungs indicates that the tube is functioning properly. The loss of lung sounds on either side is cause for immediate action.

22. B. Preschoolers use dramatic play to act out the drama of life. The nurse can use fantasy play to communicate facts about asthma at the child's developmental level.

CASE STUDIES

1. A. Learn apnea monitor operation, maintenance, and troubleshooting. If the apnea alarm sounds and the infant is not breathing, stimulate the infant's back or feet. Proceed to more vigorous stimulation if needed. (Do *not* shake the infant vigrously. This could cause additional serious injuries.) If the infant does not respond, begin cardiopulmonary resuscitation (CPR) and call the emergency rescue squad.
   B. Encourage CPR and Heimlich maneuver training.
   C. Notify telephone and electrical companies of the use of the monitor in the home.
   D. Keep emergency numbers by all phones.

2. Drooling is a characteristic symptom of epiglottitis. Avoid placing anything in the child's mouth, since this can cause laryngospasm. Keep the child as calm as possible.

ALTERATIONS IN CARDIOVASCULAR FUNCTION

Chapter Overview

Chapter 12 focuses on alterations in cardiovascular function that may result from congenital defects, acquired infections causing damage to the heart, vascular diseases, and injury to the heart muscle from trauma. The transition from fetal to pulmonary circulation is described, and normal pediatric differences in cardiovascular function are presented. Etiology, symptoms, and treatment of congestive heart failure are discussed in detail. Acyanotic and cyanotic congenital defects are examined, and the medical and nursing management of children with these defects is presented. Home care before and after surgery is also described. Acquired and vascular diseases and injuries to the cardiovascular system are also discussed.

Learning Objectives

After studying this chapter, you should be able to:
- Compare the fetal and pulmonary circulation of the heart.
- Describe changes that occur in three fetal cardiovascular structures after birth.
- Discuss the child's response to chronic hypoxemia.
- Describe the etiology and clinical manifestations of congestive heart failure (CHF) and the medical and nursing management of children with this disorder.
- Differentiate between cyanotic and acyanotic heart defects.
- Discuss the anatomy and clinical manifestations of selected acyanotic heart defects and the medical and nursing management of children with these defects.
- Discuss the anatomy and clinical manifestations of cyanotic heart defects and the clinical and nursing management of children with these defects.
- Outline the diagnostic tests and procedures used to diagnose congenital heart diseases.
- Discuss the etiology of selected cardiac and vascular diseases and the medical and nursing management of children with these diseases.
- Discuss the etiology of selected injuries to the cardiovascular system and the medical and nursing management of children with these injuries.

Review of Concepts

MATCHING

Match the items in list 1 with the appropriate word or phrase in list 2.

1. Congenital Heart Defects

LIST 1
A. Acyanotic defect
B. Cyanotic defect

LIST 2
1. _____ Ventricular septal defect
2. _____ Patent ductus arteriosus
3. _____ Tetralogy of Fallot
4. _____ Coarctation of the aorta
5. _____ Transposition of the great vessels
6. _____ Hypoplastic left heart

2. Cardiac Shunts

LIST 1
A. Right-to-left shunt
B. Left-to-right shunt

LIST 2
1. _____ Atrial septal defect
2. _____ Tetralogy of Fallot
3. _____ Transposition of the great vessels
4. _____ Patent ductus arteriosus
5. _____ Ventricular septal defect
6. _____ Hypoplastic left heart

SHORT ESSAY

1. Describe the factors that cause the foramen ovale and ductus arteriosus to close after birth.

2. A 2-year-old child has a heart rate of 190 beats/min. What is significant about this heart rate?

3. The chest x-ray film of an infant with pneumonia reveals that the heart is enlarged. What is the significance of this finding?

4. List signs of digoxin toxicity.

5. How do cyanotic heart defects differ from acyanotic heart defects?

6. Describe the mechanics of a left-to-right shunt and a right-to-left shunt in congenital heart disease.

7. Describe postoperative care for a child after repair of a heart defect.

8. Describe the basic discharge instructions for a child after repair of an acyanotic heart defect.

9. Describe the symptoms that occur with infective endocarditis.

Critical Thinking: Application/Analysis

MULTIPLE CHOICE

Select the best answer.

1. Which of the following is a characteristic physiologic response in children to a state of chronic hypoxemia?

   A. Congestive heart failure
   B. Tachycardia
   C. Polycythemia
   D. Anemia

2. An early symptom of CHF in an infant is:

   A. Wheezing
   B. Tiring easily
   C. Tachypnea
   D. Cyanosis

3. When CHF is well controlled, the child's:

   A. Diuretic dose can be decreased
   B. Energy level is increased
   C. Heart rate will be normal
   D. Digoxin dose can be decreased

4. The newborn heart increases cardiac output by:

   A. Increasing heart rate
   B. Decreasing heart rate
   C. Distention of ventricles
   D. Expansion of atria

5. Cardiac arrest in children generally results from:

   A. Hypercholesterolemia
   B. Prolonged tachycardia
   C. Myocardial infarction
   D. Prolonged hypoxemia

6. Digoxin overdose is more common when the child's:

   A. Activity level is increased
   B. Diuretic dose is reduced
   C. Potassium level is reduced
   D. Fluid intake is reduced

7. The position of choice to facilitate oxygenation in a child on bedrest is:

   A. Flat
   B. Semi-Fowler
   C. Trendelenberg
   D. High Fowler

8. A strategy to improve nutrition in an infant who tires easily is to feed the infant:

   A. Every hour
   B. Every 6 hours
   C. Solid foods
   D. High-calorie formula

9. The symptoms that result from a patent ductus arteriosus are directly related to the:

   A. Flow of oxygenated blood back into pulmonary artery
   B. Flow of unoxygenated blood into aorta from pulmonary artery
   C. Decrease in volume of oxygenated blood entering left atrium
   D. Flow of oxygenated blood into systemic circulation

10. Pulmonic stenosis causes:

   A. Left ventricular hypertrophy
   B. Right ventricular hypertrophy
   C. Pulmonary hypertension
   D. Left-to-right shunt

11. A physical assessment finding that may indicate coarctation of the aorta is:

   A. Low blood pressure in arms
   B. High blood pressure in legs
   C. Weak femoral pulses
   D. Weak radial pulses

12. The first symptom of an acyanotic heart defect is often:

   A. Cyanosis
   B. Poor weight gain
   C. Tachypnea
   D. Heart murmur

13. The surgical procedure used to correct pulmonic stenosis is:

   A. Valvuloplasty
   B. Transcatheter closure
   C. Mustard/Senning
   D. Pulmonary artery banding

14. After a cardiac catheterization, the plan of care would include:

   A. Applying direct pressure over site for 1 hour
   B. Encouraging activity after 2 hours
   C. Encouraging fluid intake
   D. Maintaining NPO status for 6 hours

15. A simple, noninvasive method to assess adequacy of tissue perfusion is:

   A. Echocardiography
   B. Capillary refill
   C. Serum electrolyte monitoring
   D. Arterial blood gas monitoring

16. An unexplained fever or malaise seen within the 2 months after repair of a heart defect may indicate:

   A. Infective endocarditis
   B. Simple cold or flu
   C. Infected incision
   D. Pneumonia

17. Which of the following is a common manifestation of chronic hypoxemia?

   A. Slow respiratory rate
   B. Low hematocrit and hemoglobin
   C. Capillary refill less than 2 seconds
   D. Clubbing of fingers and toes

18. The severity of symptoms in tetralogy of Fallot is determined by:

    A. Amount of blood that enters aorta
    B. Size of ventricular septal defect
    C. Degree of pulmonic stenosis
    D. Presence of atrial septal defect

19. Survival of a newborn with transposition of the great vessels depends on:

    A. Minimal obstruction of pulmonary artery
    B. Continued patency of ductus arteriosus and foramen ovale
    C. Proper closure of ductus arteriosus
    D. Dilation of pulmonary vessels

20. Signs of complications from polycythemia include headache, dizziness, and:

    A. Paralysis
    B. Warm, moist skin
    C. Chest pain
    D. Brisk capillary refill

21. A characteristic position assumed by a toddler with tetralogy of Fallot is:

    A. Trendelenberg
    B. Supine
    C. Squatting
    D. Sitting with head forward

22. When a child with a cyanotic heart defect has a cyanotic episode, the initial treatment is to calm the child, give oxygen, and place the child in a:

    A. Reverse Trendelenberg position
    B. Knee–chest position
    C. High Fowler position
    D. Supine position

23. Infants with cyanotic heart disease are often difficult to feed because of:

    A. Poor suck and swallow reflexes
    B. Apneic episodes and sleepiness
    C. Poor appetite and low caloric needs
    D. Dyspnea and fatigue

24. Children with polycythemia are at risk if they develop:

    A. Headaches
    B. Dehydration
    C. Cold symptoms
    D. Constipation

25. Which of the following methods can be used to reduce the heart rate in children experiencing supraventricular tachycardia?

    A. Apply ice to face
    B. Place in Trendelenberg position
    C. Induce hyperventilation
    D. Perform precordial thump

26. The incidence of rheumatic fever can be reduced by:

    A. Culturing and treating strep throat infections
    B. Giving all contacts antibiotics
    C. Isolating children with rheumatic fever
    D. Immunizing children against disease

27. Discharge instructions for a child with rheumatic fever need to emphasize compliance with:

    A. Monthly throat cultures
    B. Daily exercise regimen
    C. Long-term antibiotic treatment
    D. Serial electrocardiograms every year

28. A condition that places children at risk for infective endocardia is:

    A. Hypercholesterolemia
    B. Congenital heart defects
    C. Migraine headaches
    D. Sinus tachycardia

29. Children with Kawasaki disease often receive aspirin for:

    A. Control of pain
    B. Reduction of inflammation
    C. Antithrombolytic therapy
    D. Long-term control of fever

30. Hyperlipidemia can be managed in most children by:

    A. Weight loss
    B. Antihypertensive medication
    C. Digoxin and furosemide (Lasix)
    D. Diet and exercise

31. One test that can monitor the progress in treating hypovolemic shock is hourly:

    A. Blood replacement
    B. Serum potassium level
    C. Arterial blood gases
    D. Urine specific gravity

32. Myocardial contusion should be suspected in a motor vehicle accident in which:

    A. Car was struck from behind
    B. Shoulder straps abraded chest and neck
    C. Child is ejected from vehicle
    D. Driver's chest hits steering wheel

CASE STUDIES

1. Jamal, 14 months old, may have a congenital heart defect. He has a heart murmur, has had several respiratory infections, and is growing very slowly. Describe for his parents the diagnostic tests he will undergo.

2. Parents of 10-day-old Kathleen, who has been diagnosed with tetralogy of Fallot, are concerned that their infant will be undergoing surgery at such a young age. What information would you give Kathleen's parents about the benefits of early intervention in this condition?

3. Ryan, 10 years old, was riding his bicycle when he fell, striking his abdomen and rib cage with the handle bars. He was brought to the hospital by his parents when they noticed that he was pale, his arms were cool, his heart was beating rapidly, and he had abdominal pain. Ryan was diagnosed with hypovolemic shock resulting from a ruptured spleen. How would you explain this diagnosis to his parents?

Suggested Learning Activities

1. Contact the local chapter of the American Heart Association. Investigate the following areas:
    A. What services are available to families of a child with a congenital heart defect?
    B. Are families referred to parent support groups?
    C. What educational services are available for families and for the community?

2. Contact the health department in your community or region. Investigate:
    A. The types of congenital heart defects that are commonly found in your area.
    B. How the incidence of those defects in your community compares to the national average.
    C. Whether there is a higher than expected rate of occurrence of heart defects, and, if so, whether any environmental conditions (e.g., pollution, natural uranium veins) could be implicated in this increased incidence.

ANSWERS WITH RATIONALES

Review of Concepts

MATCHING

1.   1. A   2. A   3. B
        4. A   5. B   6. B

2.   1. B   2. A   3. A
        4. B   5. B   6. A

SHORT ESSAY

1. The foramen ovale, an opening between the atria in the fetal heart, allows most of the oxygenated blood to bypass the pulmonary circulation and flow directly from the right atrium to the left atrium, and then out to the systemic circulation. In utero, the lungs are filled with fluid; therefore pulmonary vascular resistance is high. Because the pulmonary vessels are constricted, the pulmonary circulation is limited. The systemic vascular resistance is low, enabling blood to flow easily to the extremities. When the umbilical cord is clamped, the systemic vascular resistance rises, causing a backup of blood flow, and resulting in an increase in pressure on the left side of the heart. This stimulates the foramen ovale to close.

   The ductus arteriosus in the fetus shunts blood from the pulmonary artery to the aorta and the systemic circulation. When breathing begins, the lungs become air filled, and pulmonary resistance falls. With the rise in systemic vascular resistance, blood no longer flows into the aorta through the ductus arteriosus. The ductus responds to the higher oxygen saturation that occurs as a result of the more efficient pulmonary circulation, normally constricting and closing within 10 to 15 hours after birth. Permanent closure occurs by 10 to 21 days after birth. If the oxygen saturation remains low, the ductus may stay open, allowing the flow of unoxygenated blood into the systemic circulation.

2. When the heart rate reaches 180 beats/min in a child (220 beats/min in an infant), there is not enough time for blood to fill the ventricles during diastole. The cardiac output and stroke volume decrease, and shock leading to death may develop if the heart rate is not reduced.

3. Several congenital heart defects disrupt the flow of blood through the heart, lungs, or aorta. When the flow to one area is restricted (e.g., the pulmonary artery is narrowed), the work of the heart is increased. This causes the ventricle that is working harder to enlarge or hypertrophy. Initially blood flow increases; however, the heart eventually fails. Therefore an enlarged heart on a chest x-ray is an indication to evaluate the child for a congenital or acquired heart defect.

4. Signs of digoxin toxicity include:
   A. Bradycardia (<100 beats/min in a young child, <80 beats/min in an older child, and <60 beats/min in an adolescent)
   B. Arrhythmia
   C. Dizziness, headache
   D. Weakness, fatigue

5. Heart defects are classified as either cyanotic or acyanotic; however, this classification is misleading because clinical cyanosis can be present with both types. Cyanotic defects are those in which unoxygenated blood is pumped into the systemic circulation and cyanosis occurs frequently. Acyanotic defects are those in which oxygenated blood is shunted back into the pulmonary artery, causing excess fluid volume to flow through the pul-

monary vascular system. The child may appear cyanotic when pulmonary vascular resistance develops and unoxygenated blood begins to flow away from the pulmonary artery into the left side of the heart and from there to the systemic circulation. Thus, classification is based on the hemodynamics originally seen in the heart.

6. A shunt is the movement of blood through an abormal opening between the chambers of the heart. The opening may be between ventricles, atria, or major vessels in the heart. The right side of the heart pumps blood into the pulmonary system, and the left side pumps blood through the aorta into the body. Blood flows from areas of high pressure to areas of low pressure. The blood in the left side of the heart is under higher presure because the force needed to pump blood into the body is much higher. When there is a hole between the ventricles, the higher pressure on the left side initially causes the blood to flow from the left ventricle to the right ventricle, resulting in blood that is already oxygenated flowing back into the pulmonary system. This is an example of a left-to-right shunt, which leads to pulmonary system overload. This overload can result in pulmonary vascular resistance, causing an increase in the force needed to pump blood into the pulmonary vessels. As the pulmonary resistance increases, the pressure in the right side of the heart rises until the pressure on the right side is higher than that on the left side. This causes the blood to flow through the opening from the right ventricle to the left ventricle, allowing unoxygenated blood to be pumped into the body. This is an example of a right-to-left shunt. If not enough blood is oxygenated, cyanosis results.

7. The child is transferred to the pediatric intensive care unit immediately after repair of a heart defect and may require intubation and ventilation for a short time. During this period, assessments include monitoring of vital signs, measuring intake and output, monitoring the level of consciousness and heart function, and checking for arrhythmias. In addition, it is necessary to check for hemorrhage, adequate ventilation and tissue perfusion, and acid–base and electrolyte imbalances.

Once the child returns to a general nursing unit, the focus of assessment shifts to monitoring for com-plications of surgery such as infections, arrhythmias, and impaired tissue perfusion. Monitor the incision site for signs of infection, which include spreading erythema, drainage, and increased pain. Assess the lungs carefully for breath sounds, respiratory effort, and signs of distress, which may indicate pneumonia or fluid accumulation in the lungs or pleural space. Check for arrhythmias, which can be recognized by an irregular heart beat or bradycardia when taking apical pulses. These must be reported immediately, because they indicate reduced cardiac output, which requires correction. Monitor tissue perfusion by checking capillary refill, extremity warmth, pedal pulses, level of consciousness, and urine output. Decreased urinary output is another sign of reduced cardiac output, which must be corrected.

8. Discharge instructions for a child after repair of an acyanotic heart defect should include:
   A. Allowing a gradual increase in activity as tolerated by the child and reporting any significant changes in activity level to the physician.
   B. Observing for and reporting any of the following signs of infection: fever; erythema around incision, drainage, or increased pain (signs of a wound infection); flulike symptoms; increased respiratory rate; or respiratory distress.
   C. Allowing the child to return to school in 3 weeks, and to resume all normal activities in 6 weeks.

9. Symptoms of infective endocarditis can be mild and develop slowly, or they can be severe and develop rapidly. Symptoms include fever (with afternoon elevations), fatigue, joint and muscle aches, headache, gastrointestinal discomfort, chest pain, dyspnea, weight loss, splenomegaly, and arrhythmias or murmurs.

Critical Thinking: Application/Analysis

MULTIPLE CHOICE

1. C. In chronic hypoxemia, the body attempts to make more hemoglobin available to carry oxygen by producing more red blood cells, which results

in polycythemia. If the concentration of red blood cells becomes too high (hematocrit greater than 55% to 60%), the blood becomes thick and viscous, placing the child at risk for thromboembolism. Polycythemia is common in children with cyanotic heart defects.

2. B. Early signs of CHF are subtle and often missed. Tiring easily, particularly during feeding, is one sign during infancy.

3. B. When CHF is controlled, the oxygen flow to the tissues improves, which increases the child's energy level. The child begins to develop normally again because the physiologic threat is decreased.

4. A. The newborn heart is not able to increase stroke volume; thus the only way to increase cardiac output is to increase the heart rate.

5. D. Cardiac arrests in infants and children are related to hypoxemia that is a result of respiratory failure or shock, rather than a primary cardiac insult as in adults. Bradycardia is a significant warning sign of cardiac arrest.

6. C. Digoxin overdose is more common when serum potassium levels are low. Many children with heart disease receive diuretics as well as digoxin. One group of diuretics, potassium-wasting diuretics, causes potassium to be excreted in higher amounts. Caution is necessary whenever a child is receiving these potassium-wasting drugs. Potassium levels must be checked frequently to avoid digoxin overdose.

7. B. A 45-degree angle (semi-Fowler position) is the best position in which to place a child to facilitate maximum oxygenation.

8. D. Higher-calorie formulas, designed for premature infants, deliver more calories in a smaller volume. (Normal formulas have 20 cal/oz, whereas "premie" formulas have 24 cal/oz.) These formulas can help to deliver adequate nutrition in the infant who tires easily during feeding.

9. A. The ductus arteriosus allows blood to flow from the pulmonary artery into the aorta before birth. The pressure is lower in the aorta than in the pulmonary artery because the lungs are filled with fluid. After birth, the pressure gradients are reversed, and the blood in the aorta is under higher pressure, causing it to flow through the ductus into the pulmonary artery. This extra blood entering the pulmonary system can lead to CHF.

10. B. Stenosis (narrowing) of the pulmonary artery valve makes it more difficult for blood to enter the pulmonary artery, causing increased pressure within the right ventricle. This leads to right ventricular hypertrophy, because the ventricle must pump harder to move the blood into the artery.

11. C. Coarctation is a narrowing that occurs in the descending aorta. Blood flow to the legs is decreased, and flow to the arms and head is increased. The femoral pulses are weak, and the radial pulses are full.

12. D. In several of the acyanotic heart defects, blood flows under pressure across a shunt or through a narrowed vessel or valve. This turbulence creates a sound that is heard outside the heart as a murmur. The placement of the murmur may help identify the type of defect present.

13. A. Valvuloplasty improves the function of the pulmonary valve by dilating the valve with a balloon during cardiac catheterization or cardiac surgery.

14. C. The contrast medium used during a cardiac catheterization causes diuresis, so maintaining hydration is important.

15. B. Capillary refill assesses the amount of time needed for the blood to return to the tissue that has been blanched (see Chapter 3). The best site to assess refill in infants is the sole of the foot; in older children, the fingernails and toenails are preferred. The longer it takes for blood to return to the blanched area (>3 sec), the poorer

the tissue perfusion. This test is quick and painless and is a good indicator of tissue perfusion.

16. A. After cardiac surgery, children are at risk of infective endocarditis, especially within the first 6 months after surgery. They should receive prophylactic antibiotics, particularly before any dental work or invasive procedures.

17. D. Chronic hypoxemia results in clubbing of fingers and toes. The ends of the digits enlarge and become bulbous in shape. Clubbing may occur at any age.

18. C. Pulmonic stenosis is a narrowing or malfunction of the pulmonic valve, causing a decrease in the flow of blood to the lungs. The more severe the stenosis, the more severe the symptoms of hypoxemia and cyanosis.

19. B. In transposition of the great vessels, the positions of the aorta and pulmonary artery are reversed. This results in two independent circulatory systems. The aorta is the outflow for the right ventricle, and the pulmonary artery is the outflow for the left ventricle. Blood is pumped back into the body from the right ventricle without completing the pulmonary circuit; thus it is unoxygenated. Blood that is pumped into the pulmonary circuit and returns to the left ventricle is then pumped into the pulmonary artery again, so the oxygenated blood never reaches the body. To sustain life, there must be a way for the oxygenated blood to mix with the unoxygenated blood. A patent ductus arteriosus and foramen ovale allow for some mixing but can only sustain life for a short period of time. Palliative surgery is performed within a week to create a large hole between the atria that enables sufficient intermixing of oxygenated and unoxygenated blood. Corrective surgery to switch the arteries may be performed later.

20. A. Polycythemia, which is caused by increased red blood cell production, results in a high red blood cell count and thick, viscous blood. This predisposes the child to thromboembolism, which may cause stroke and paralysis.

21. C. Children with cyanotic heart defects often squat down in a knee–chest position to relieve dyspnea.

22. B. The knee–chest position reduces the cardiac output by decreasing the venous return from the lower extremities and by increasing the systemic vascular resistance. This results in an increase in pulmonary blood flow.

23. D. Infants with cyanotic heart disease tire easily because of a lack of oxygen. This lack of oxygen also results in dyspnea with exertion as the body attempts to increase oxygen levels in the blood by increasing the respiratory rate. The infant is therefore unable to suck well, resulting in inadequate nutrition and retarded growth.

24. B. Polycythemia results in an elevated hematocrit, and any degree of dehydration will cause the blood to become even more viscous. Dehydration can occur very quickly in children with vomiting and diarrhea.

25. A. Applying ice or iced saline solution to the face causes vagal stimulation that may reduce the heart rate. An older child can perform the Valsalva maneuver to increase intrathoracic and venous pressures, thus slowing the heart rate.

26. A. Rheumatic fever follows an infection with some strains of group A ß-hemolytic streptococci. Prevention focuses on obtaining cultures for all children with possible strep throat infections and, if the culture is positive, treating them with antibiotics for 10 days.

27. C. On discharge, a daily low-dose antibiotic is prescribed or a monthly long-acting antibiotic injection is given. This treatment may be indefinite, and the family must understand the importance of preventing future strep infections, and that heart damage can result from recurrent rheumatic fever.

28. B. Bacteria in the blood are usually filtered by the capillaries in the lungs. However, in cyanotic heart defects with a right-to-left shunt, some of the blood does not enter the pulmonary circuit and the bacteria remain in the blood stream. This can result in infective endocarditis.

29. C. Children with Kawasaki disease develop thrombocytosis, which places them at risk of thromboembolism. Aspirin is given until the platelet count returns to normal.

30. D. The child's diet is examined and reduction in fat content is recommended. Saturated fats are decreased, as is the total fat content of the diet. Dietary modification is advised for the entire family, because it is difficult for only one member to change his or her eating pattern and the entire family can benefit. Activity level is also examined, and aerobic exercise is recommended at least 3 times weekly.

31. D. Urine output decreases and may cease in children with hypovolemic shock because of the decreased circulation to the kidneys. An increase in urinary output and a decrease in specific gravity results are signs that the child's condition is improving.

32. D. When the driver hits the steering wheel, the blunt force against the anterior chest wall can injure the heart by disrupting blood flow to the heart muscle. This is a potentially life-threatening condition.

CASE STUDIES

1. The following tests are used in the diagnosis of congenital heart defects:
   A. A *chest x-ray* is performed to determine the size and shape of the heart. Some heart defects make the heart work harder, causing the heart muscle to become larger. This may be visible on the x-ray. The x-ray can also show whether the blood vessels in the lungs are large and congested with blood (a consequence of some types of heart defects).
   B. An *electrocardiogram* is performed to measure the electrical system in the heart. Every muscle has nerves that carry an electrical "charge" to make the muscle work. The heart has a number of nerves that send the electrical "charge" to different parts of the heart muscle. If something has interfered with the electrical pathway, the heart cannot beat normally. This test is not painful.
   C. An *echocardiogram* uses sound waves to outline the structures of the heart and the path of blood flow through the different parts of the heart. It is performed to identify the presence of an abnormality such as a hole between the chambers. This test is not painful.
   D. *Cardiac catheterization* is performed when more precise information is needed about a defect. The four chambers inside the heart normally maintain a certain amount of pressure to pump blood to the next chamber or body part. A catheter is inserted in the groin and is threaded up to the heart. The physician can watch the catheter on a special x-ray machine as it approaches and enters the heart. A sample of blood can be removed from different chambers to determine how much oxygen is in the blood in each chamber. The catheter can also accurately measure the pressure in each chamber. Defects in the heart can easily be seen when dye is squirted into one chamber of the heart. As the heart beats, the blood containing the dye is pumped through the heart. Any defect or hole is seen immediately by the movement of the dyed blood. This test is performed only with sedation or anesthesia in children because it is painful.

2. Children with cyanotic heart defects have lower levels of oxygen in their blood. Over time, this has an adverse effect on the child's mental and physical development. The low oxygen level also can cause damage to the heart, lungs, and brain. To prevent this damage, palliative surgery may be performed early in infancy to increase the oxygen levels. Corrective surgery may then be performed when the child is older.

3. Hypovolemic shock is a state of shock caused by low blood volume (e.g., from heavy bleeding). When Ryan fell, the handlebars from his bicycle struck his abdomen and lower left rib cage. The spleen, which is located in this area, is fragile and can easily rupture, resulting in heavy bleeding into the abdomen. As Ryan was losing blood, his body was trying to keep his blood circulating to vital organs such as the brain and lungs. Less blood was pumped to the arms and legs, which is why they felt cool and clammy. Ryan's heart started beating faster to try to maintain normal blood pressure and tissue oxygen levels. These were the symptoms you noticed. Had bleeding continued, Ryan's body would have been unable to keep up with the decreasing volume of blood, and a life-threatening situation would have developed. Fortunately, Ryan was brought to the hospital while his body was still able to keep his blood circulating. His treatment will begin with steps to control the bleeding in the spleen and replace the lost volume of blood.

13

ALTERATIONS IN HEMATOLOGIC FUNCTION

Chapter Overview

Chapter 13 focuses on several disorders that result in alterations in hematologic function. The normal anatomy and physiology of the hematologic system of children is presented. Disorders are grouped in two general categories: those that result in anemia and those that involve clotting defects. The medical and nursing management of each disorder is outlined, and the chapter concludes with a discussion of bone marrow transplantation for various immune diseases.

Learning Objectives

After studying this chapter, you should be able to:
- Distinguish among the cells that make up the cellular portion of blood.
- Describe how sickle cell anemia is transmitted.
- Discuss the mechanism whereby the red blood cells become sickle-shaped in sickle cell anemia.
- Differentiate among the types of sickle cell crises.
- Outline the nursing management of a child in sickle cell crisis.
- Discuss the nursing management of the populations at risk for iron deficiency anemia.
- Describe the clinical manifestations of ß-thalassemia and aplastic anemia and the medical and nursing management of children with these disorders.
- Describe how hemophilia is transmitted.
- Discuss the clinical manifestations of hemophilia and other selected clotting disorders and the medical and nursing management of children with these disorders.
- Describe bone marrow transplantation and identify conditions for which it may be used.

Review of Concepts

MATCHING

Match the items in list 1 with the appropriate word or phrase in list 2. (*Note:* Items may be used more than once.)

1. Sickle Cell Crises

LIST 1
A. Vaso-occlusive crises
B. Splenic sequestration
C. Aplastic crises

1. ____ Profound anemia
2. ____ Pooling of blood in spleen
3. ____ Decreased production of red blood cells
4. ____ Ischemia and infarction
5. ____ Death can occur in hours
6. ____ Most common type
7. ____ Triggered by viral infection
8. ____ Pain

2. Analgesics

List 1

A. Autosomal dominant trait
B. Sex-linked recessive trait
C. Autosomal recessive trait

List 2

1. ____ Hemophilia
2. ____ Sickle cell anemia
3. ____ Congenital aplastic anemia
4. ____ Von Willebrand disease
5. ____ ß-Thalassemia

Short Essay

1. Describe how the sickling process occurs in children with sickle cell anemia.

2. Discuss the pathophysiology of a vaso-occlusive sickle cell crisis.

3. Describe how sickle cell crises can be prevented.

4. List the basic defects that cause the clinical manifestations of ß-thalassemia.

5. Describe factors that place an adolescent girl at risk for developing iron deficiency anemia, and the recommended treatment.

6. Discuss patient education for a child taking an iron preparation.

Critical Thinking: Application/Analysis

Multiple Choice

Select the best answer.

1. When a blood transfusion is administered, a critical period in which to observe for adverse reactions is:

   A. 24 hours after transfusion
   B. At beginning of transfusion
   C. During second transfusion
   D. At end of transfusion

2. The major cause of death in sickle cell anemia is:

   A. Liver failure
   B. Stroke
   C. Infection
   D. Heart attack

3. Which of the following places a child with sickle cell anemia at greatest risk for a sickle cell crisis?

   A. General anesthesia
   B. Train travel
   C. Visiting large city
   D. Swimming in pool

4. Infants with sickle cell anemia rarely show any symptoms before 4 months of age because:

   A. Maternal hemoglobin does not sickle
   B. Hemoglobin S is made after 8 months
   C. Infants are rarely ill in first 4 months
   D. Fetal hemoglobin resists sickling

5. In order for a child to develop sickle cell anemia:

   A. One parent must have sickle cell anemia
   B. Both parents must have sickle cell trait
   C. One parent must have sickle cell trait
   D. A defect in cell division must occur

6. During warm weather, a child with sickle cell anemia must:

   A. Avoid any exertion
   B. Take aspirin to avoid blood clots
   C. Take corticosteroids
   D. Maintain appropriate hydration

7. Children at high risk for iron deficiency anemia are:

   A. Vegetarians who eat large amounts of raisins, nuts, and eggs
   B. Infants over 6 months of age who are fed only breast milk
   C. School-aged children who refuse to eat fruits
   D. Adolescents who eat fish but no meats

8. A child with thalassemia minor or thalassemia trait has which of the following symptoms?

   A. Thrombocytopenia
   B. Mild anemia
   C. Moderate anemia
   D. Leukopenia

9. Children with thalassemia intermedia or major are treated with blood transfusions. However, a complication of this treatment is:

   A. Polycythemia
   B. Hemosiderosis
   C. Thrombocytopenia
   D. Iron deficiency

10. ß-Thalassemia is an inherited blood disorder found most often in people of:

   A. Scandinavian descent
   B. North American descent
   C. Mediterranean descent
   D. Native American descent

11. The treatment of choice for children with aplastic anemia is:

   A. Bone marrow transplantation
   B. Liver transplantation
   C. Iron supplementation
   D. Serial blood transfusions

12. Persons with aplastic anemia are at risk for bleeding because of:

   A. Polycythemia
   B. Neutropenia
   C. Leukopenia
   D. Thrombocytopenia

13. Hemophilia is a sex-linked recessive trait, which means it is transmitted from:

   A. Grandfather to mother to son
   B. Grandmother to mother to son
   C. Grandfather to father to son
   D. Grandmother to father to son

14. To avoid the risk of transmission of the human immunodeficiency virus (HIV), children with mild hemophilia are often treated with:

   A. Cryoprecipitate
   B. Desmopressin (DDAVP)
   C. Fresh frozen plasma
   D. Factor VIII concentrate

15. A common characteristic of von Willebrand disease is:

   A. Abdominal bleeding
   B. Iron deficiency anemia
   C. Hemarthrosis
   D. Epistaxis

16. You notice that a child receiving a blood transfusion has developed a fever. Your first action is to:

   A. Give acetaminophen
   B. Stop infusion
   C. Notify physician
   D. Administer epinephrine

17. Children with idiopathic thrombocytopenic purpura (ITP) who do not respond to corticosteroids and immunoglobulins may have to undergo:

A. Splenectomy
B. Blood transfusion
C. Platelet transfusion
D. Bone marrow transplantation

18. After bone marrow transplantation, a child is at high risk for:

A. Marrow rejection
B. Dehydration
C. Bleeding
D. Infection

CASE STUDIES

1. In the opening vignette, Michael, who is 12 years old, is in sickle cell crisis. The crisis was triggered by a viral illness. Michael is experiencing severe abdominal pain and is very anxious and frightened. Summarize the nursing care that Michael requires.

2. Fourteen-month-old Shuja has been walking for 2 months. He has a history of easy bruising and began limping after a fall in his front yard. His physical examination revealed a swollen, tender left knee and multiple bruises along his arms and legs. He-mophilia A has been diagnosed after discovery of a deficiency of factor VIII in Shuja's blood. This diagnosis is a surprise to his parents, because there is no history of hemophilia in the family. Outline a nursing management plan for Shuja.

Suggested Learning Activities

1. Contact a genetic counselor who has experience with families who carry the sickle cell trait.
   A. What testing is done when parents are referred?
   B. What counseling is given to these couples?
   C. Are referrals made to other organizations or support groups?

2. Visit a hospital where bone marrow transplantation is performed. Tour the unit and note the types of isolation rooms used for these patients. Some areas to investigate are:
   A. How do staff meet the developmental needs of children who are in strict isolation?
   B. What support systems are in place for parents and family members?
   C. What is the total cost of bone marrow transplantation? What percentage of this cost is covered by insurance?

ANSWERS WITH RATIONALES

Review of Concepts

MATCHING

1.

1. B, C	2. B	3. C
4. A	5. B	6. A
7. C	8. A	

2.

1. B	2. C	3. C
4. A	5. C	

SHORT ESSAY

1. In children with sickle cell anemia, normal hemoglobin A is replaced by an abnormal variant called hemoglobin S. Under certain conditions hemoglobin S changes its crystalline shape, causing the red blood cell it is part of to become elongated and assume a crescent shape with two pointed ends. The conditions that can cause this change are increased blood viscosity (from fever, dehydration, or poor fluid intake) and hypoxia or low oxygen tension (from high altitudes, vasoconstriction when cold, or an emotionally stressful event).

2. In a vaso-occlusive crisis, a significant number of red blood cells are triggered by some factor (fever, infection, emotional stress, etc.) to assume a sickle shape. Normally the round shape of the red blood cell allows it to slip easily through the vast complex of veins and arteries. However, the sickle-shaped cells are rigid and become entangled in the capillaries, causing an obstruction to capillary blood flow. This obstruction leads to engorgement or stasis of blood, tissue ischemia, and ultimately tissue hypoxia, which results in large infarctions. The damaged tissues are often located in vital organs, which become scarred, resulting in impaired fuction. Damage to the spleen is common, resulting in impaired func-

tion of the child's immune system. The sickled cells can resume their normal shape, if undamaged, when they are reoxygenated and rehydrated. They are, however, very fragile and have a greatly shortened life span, 10 to 20 days, as opposed to 120 days for unsickled cells. Because the sickled red blood cells are easily damaged, the bone marrow continually produces more blood cells. However, children with frequent sickle cell crises often have severe hemolytic anemia.

3. Prevention of sickling episodes focuses on maintaining normal oxygenation and hydration. Avoiding infections is also important because fever and dehydration, which often accompany infection, are common triggers. Avoiding activities or situations in which the oxygenation status can be compromised is also vital. Examples of these situations include extreme physical exertion, land travel at high altitude, travel in poorly pressurized airplanes, hypoventilation, and emotionally stressful events. It is important to make appropriate travel plans and to avoid extremes of exercise and stress, if possible.

4. The basic defects in ß-thalassemia are:
   A. Defective synthesis of hemoglobin
   B. Structurally impaired red blood cells
   C. Shortened life span of red blood cells

5. Adolescents are in a growth spurt for several years. This rapid growth places high nutritional demands on the body, and the teen needs adequate iron stores for optimal growth. During this developmental stage the peer group is very important. Diet is often determined by the group and may be very unbalanced. Many teenage girls place themselves on strict reducing diets that contain little or no iron. Girls also begin to menstruate at puberty, which results in additional iron loss. Dietary management with iron supplementation is the preferred method of treat-

ment. Emphasizing the benefits of treatment (better skin color, more energy, improvement in growth) may increase compliance.

6. Elemental iron is given to reverse iron deficiency anemia. The liquid preparations can stain the teeth, so they need to be sipped through a straw. The presence of black, tarry stools indicates that sufficient iron is being ingested. Side effects include the black stools, constipation, and a foul aftertaste to the preparation. A diet high in iron is advised in addition to the iron supplement.

Critical Thinking: Application/Analysis

MULTIPLE CHOICE

1. B. A blood reaction can occur as soon as the transfusion begins. Therefore, administer the first 20 mL of blood slowly, observing for reaction during this time, and repeat assessments throughout the transfusion.

2. C. The major cause of death is from infection, because the nonfunctioning spleen places the child in an immunocompromised state.

3. A. Hypoxia resulting from general anesthesia is a major surgical risk. Sickle cell crisis could begin during surgery, placing this patient at high risk. Special precautions must be taken before any surgery. Therefore, it is necessary that children with sickle cell anemia be appropriately identified prior to surgery.

4. D. Fetal hemoglobin is produced throughout gestation and, at birth, is contained in all of the infant's red blood cells. After birth the infant begins to produce nonfetal hemoglobin. The normal life span of a red blood cell is 120 days. Therefore, after 4 months nearly all of the red blood cells that were present at birth have been broken down, and new cells with nonfetal hemoglobin have replaced them. In the child with sickle cell anemia the new cells contain hemoglobin S, leaving the child vulnerable to sickle cell crises.

5. B. Sickle cell anemia is an autosomal recessive disorder (see box). Each parent must carry the trait in order to produce a child with sickle cell anemia. There is a 25% risk with each pregnancy.

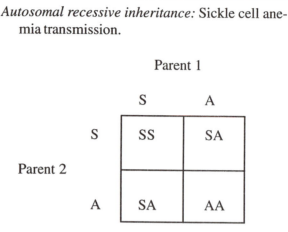

Autosomal recessive inheritance: Sickle cell anemia transmission.

	Parent 1	
	S	A
S	SS	SA
A	SA	AA

Parent 2

SS = Sickle cell anemia — 25% risk
SA = Sickle cell trait — 50% risk
AA = Normal hemoglobin — 25% risk

Note:
- If one parent has the disease and one has the trait, there is a 50% risk with each pregnancy of having a child with the disease and a 50% risk for the trait.
- If both parents have the disease, 100% of their children will have the disease.
- If one parent has the disease and the other is normal, 100% of their children will have the trait.

6. D. Dehydration is a major trigger for sickle cell crisis, and fluid intake must be increased during hot weather to replace lost fluids.

7. B. By 6 months of age, neonatal iron stores are depleted. Breast milk contains some iron but not in a large enough quantity to meet the infant's iron needs. The infant needs the addition of iron-fortified foods to meet iron needs.

8. B. Thalassemia trait results in symptoms of mild anemia.

9. B. Numerous blood transfusions add extra iron to the body, causing an overload of iron in the body. The iron is not excreted; rather, it is stored in tissues and organs. This condition is known as hemosiderosis. Iron-chelating medications are given along with vitamin C to promote iron excretion.

10. C. ß-Thalassemia occurs most often in persons of Mediterranean descent. However, it is also found among persons of Middle Eastern, Asian, and African descent.

11. A. Aplastic anemia results from the failure of the bone marrow to produce adequate numbers of blood cells. Bone marrow transplantation from a compatible sibling or family member donor is the treatment of choice.

12. D. Platelets have a major role in normal blood clotting. In thrombocytopenia there is a low platelet count, which impairs the normal clotting mechanism, resulting in bleeding and hemorrhage.

13. A. The woman who inherits the trait from her father has a 50% chance of transmitting the disease to her sons and a 50% chance of transmitting the trait to her daughters (see box).

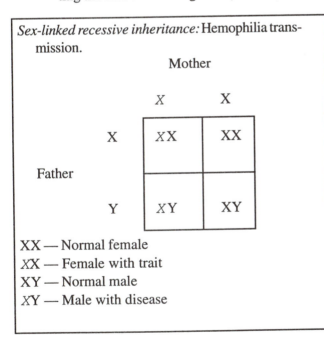

Sex-linked recessive inheritance: Hemophilia transmission.

Mother

	X	X
X	*X*X	XX
Y	*X*Y	XY

Father

XX — Normal female
*X*X — Female with trait
XY — Normal male
*X*Y — Male with disease

14. B. DDAVP is a synthetic drug that temporarily increases the activity of factor VIII two- to threefold. The chance of HIV transmission is eliminated, because the drug is synthetic and thus contains no human blood components.

15. D. Epistaxis and easy bruising are characteristic manifestations of von Willebrand disease.

16. B. Fever is a sign of blood transfusion reaction, and the infusion must be stopped immediately, even before the physician is notified. To keep the IV line open, change to a normal saline solution infusion.

17. A. In ITP the platelets are destroyed faster than they are produced by the bone marrow. The spleen is the organ that destroys the platelets. If there is no response to the drug therapy over a period of 6 months to 1 year, the spleen may be removed.

18. D. The child is without immunity for a minimum of 10 days after bone marrow transplantation and is at high risk for infection. The child must be kept in strict isolation during this period.

CASE STUDIES

1. The nursing care plan for this child in sickle cell crisis includes:
   A. *Increase tissue perfusion.* Give blood transfusions to decrease the blood viscosity, and add normal red blood cells to transport more oxygen to the tissues. To prevent hemolysis, blood should be warmed, and saline solution should be given intravenously before and after transfusion. Give oxygen as needed to increase oxygen levels in the tissues. Initiate measures to decrease emotional stress and physical exertion, which can cause tissue hypoxia.
   B. *Promote hydration.* All efforts to decrease or prevent dehydration need to be addressed, because dehydration can trigger sickling. Encourage oral intake of fluids, particularly when Michael is thirsty (e.g., upon resting after play). Offer a variety of drinks and use a small cup,

which is less intimidating than a large drinking glass. Have Michael keep track of how many such cupfuls are emptied, because he is old enough to assume this responsibility. Calculate Michael's optimal intake using fluid maintenance requirements (see Chapter 8). Give IV fluids as ordered and keep accurate intake and output records, to avoid dehydration.

C. *Control pain.* During a crisis, pain is often severe and analgesics need to be given around the clock. Nonanalgesic therapy includes positioning for comfort, avoiding any stress on painful joints.

D. *Prevent infection.* Children are susceptible to infection during a crisis. Isolate Michael from possible sources of infection, particularly other people. Report any signs of infection immediately.

E. *Ensure adequate nutrition.* Poor growth is a complication of sickle cell anemia, and Michael needs to be encouraged to eat a high-protein, high-calorie diet with folic acid supplements as ordered (depleted folic acid is a trigger for aplastic crisis).

F. *Prevent complications of crisis.* Observe for signs of increased anemia and shock (mental status change, pallor, vital sign changes). Assess for altered cerebral function, and administer blood transfusions.

2. The nursing management for Shuja will include:

A. *Control bleeding in the knee joint.* Bleeding is controlled by giving factor VIII replacement. The joint is immobilized and elevated, and ice is applied to promote vasoconstriction. Toddlers are normally very active, and it will be difficult to minimize Shuja's activity to decrease the strain placed on his leg. Constant supervision is necessary to ensure that weight is kept off the leg until bleeding is controlled.

B. *Limit joint involvement and manage pain.* The steps listed above will decrease the bleeding in the knee joint (hemarthrosis). The blood in the joint causes joint limitation from pain and swelling and can lead to bone changes, contractures, and disabling deformities. Analgesics are given as ordered and, once the bleeding is controlled, range of motion exercises are performed to strengthen muscles and prevent flexion contractures. The analgesics should be given orally to prevent any potential bleeding from an injection. Aspirin should be avoided because of the increased bleeding that may occur.

C. *Provide emotional support.* Shuja's family is surprised by this diagnosis, because there is no family history of hemophilia (one third of all children with hemophilia have no family members with a positive history). Encourage Shuja's parents to verbalize their feelings. Teach them about the disease, explain how bleeding occurs, and describe the usual treatment measures. Encourage genetic counseling, particularly in view of the lack of positive family history.

D. *Discharge planning and home care teaching.* Advise Shuja's parents to get a Medic–Alert bracelet for their son. This can be placed on his wrist or ankle. Teach the parents how to recognize signs of internal bleeding, and bleeding into the joints. If these signs occur or if Shuja has obvious bleeding, he will need immediate factor VIII infusion. (Because Shuja is so young, his parents will probably not be instructed in home administration of the factor concentrate. Be sure that the parents know where to go to get the factor VIII.) Shuja needs to be properly supervised and his toys need to be safe and age-appropriate; however, encourage the parents to avoid being overprotective. When he gets older, Shuja should avoid participation in contact sports, but sports such as swimming, bicycling, and hiking can be encouraged. Reinforce to his parents that any child care providers also need to be instructed in how to recognize bleeding and how to protect Shuja from trauma. Shuja's parents may also benefit from referral to the National Hemophilia Foundation.

14

ALTERATIONS IN
CELLULAR GROWTH

Chapter Overview

Chapter 14 focuses on alterations in cellular growth in children. The chapter opens with a general discussion of childhood cancer. Topics covered include differences between cancers in adults and children, treatment methods and their common side effects, and general nursing care of the child and family in the hospital and at home. Selected childhood cancers are then discussed in greater detail, including brain tumors, neuroblastoma, Wilms' tumor, bone tumors, leukemia, and soft tissue tumors.

Learning Objectives

After studying this chapter, you should be able to:
- Explain the significance of the differences between adult and pediatric cancers.
- Describe the general etiology of cancer in children.
- Discuss the various therapies used to treat childhood cancer.
- Describe the effect of a child's cancer diagnosis on the family.
- Describe the nursing assessment and management of children undergoing treatment for cancer.
- Discuss the clinical manifestations of selected childhood cancers and their medical and nursing management.

Review of Concepts

MATCHING

Match the items in list 1 with the appropriate word or phrase in list 2.

1. Terminology Related to Alterations in Cellular Growth

LIST 1
A. Benign
B. Malignant
C. Neoplasm
D. Oncogene
E. Chemotherapy
F. Radiation
G. Metastasis
H. Carcinogens

LIST 2

1. _____ Movement of cancer cells to other sites in body
2. _____ Drug treatment that kills normal and cancerous cells
3. _____ Chemicals or processes that, when combined with genetic traits and in interaction with one another, cause cancer
4. _____ Cancer treatment using unstable isotopes to destroy cells
5. _____ Growth that does not endanger life
6. _____ Portion of altered DNA that, when duplicated, causes uncontrolled cellular division
7. _____ Progressive growth of a tumor that will result in death
8. _____ Cancerous growth

2. Childhoold Malignancies and Clinical Manifestations

(*Note:* Items may be used more than once.)

LIST 1

A. Brain tumors
B. Neuroblastoma
C. Wilms' tumor
D. Osteosarcoma
E. Ewing sarcoma
F. Leukemia
G. Hodgkin's disease
H. Rhabdomyosarcoma
I. Retinoblastoma

LIST 2

1. _____ Pain and swelling of bones
2. _____ Nontender lymphadenopathy
3. _____ Extraorbital mass
4. _____ Vomiting and headache
5. _____ Nontender mass
6. _____ White pupil in eye
7. _____ Fever, signs of bleeding

SHORT ESSAY

1. What lifestyle changes have an effect on the incidence of childhood cancer?

2. Describe the five common signs of childhood cancer.

3. Describe the three goals of cancer treatment in children.

4. List five therapies that are used to treat cancer.

5. Discuss the use of protocols for cancer treatment.

6. Nausea and vomiting are common side effects of chemotherapy. Describe several nursing interventions that may help alleviate these side effects.

7. Describe the goal of bone marrow transplantation.

8. When a child is diagnosed with cancer, the family is in a state of crisis. Describe techniques that would provide support to the family at this time.

9. List three common threats to body image that children with cancer experience.

10. List support systems that may be available to help the family of a child with cancer.

11. Describe strategies to prepare students and teachers for the return of a classmate who is being treated for cancer.

12. Describe some of the long-term complications of treatment for children with brain tumors.

13. Explain why a child with leukemia commonly experiences abnormal bleeding.

Critical Thinking: Application/Analysis

MULTIPLE CHOICE

Select the best answer.

1. Chemotherapeutic drugs are most effective:

A. When given orally
B. When administered in sequence
C. During active cell division
D. Over a prolonged period

2. Anabolic androgenic steroids are:

   A. Oncogenes
   B. Carcinogens
   C. Neoplasms
   D. Immunosuppressants

3. Which of the following tissues is most sensitive to chemotherapeutic drugs?

   A. Skin
   B. Mucous membranes
   C. Muscle
   D. Nerves

4. One difficulty encountered when young children receive radiation treatments is that children:

   A. Experience more side effects than adults
   B. Are extremely sensitive to radiation
   C. Will be infertile in future
   D. Must maintain fixed position during treatment

5. A child receiving chemotherapy experiences thrombocytopenia from bone marrow suppression. The family needs to be instructed to protect the child from:

   A. Exposure to sunlight
   B. Bruising
   C. Mouth sores
   D. Dehydration

6. During periods of immune suppression the child is vulnerable to:

   A. Skin breakdown
   B. Liver dysfunction
   C. Overwhelming infection
   D. Kidney dysfunction

7. An advantage of an implanted venous access device in a child with cancer is:

   A. It allows child to participate in activities such as swimming
   B. It is permanent

C. It decreases number of chemotherapy sessions required
D. It requires no care

8. A strategy to help a child receiving chemotherapy in the hospital to maintain preadmission weight is to:

   A. Offer liquids and semisolid foods only
   B. Avoid salty foods that can sting mouth
   C. Offer familiar foods
   D. Make meal times into contest among children

9. What is the best measure to ensure that a child with cancer remains free from infection at home?

   A. Encourage proper handwashing
   B. Discourage visitation by friends
   C. Have child wear mask
   D. Sterilize toys weekly

10. Why is chemotherapy often ineffective in the treatment of brain tumors?

   A. Brain tumors grow very slowly and drugs only kill rapidly dividing cells.
   B. Blood-brain barrier keeps many drugs from entering brain.
   C. Cells in brain tumors are not as sensitive to drugs as to radiation.
   D. Brain tumors do not respond to any therapy and are usually fatal.

11. Which of the following clinical manifestations is suggestive of a brain tumor?

   A. Easy bruising
   B. Vomiting
   C. Diarrhea
   D. Fluid retention

12. An endocrine problem that is a possible complication of brain surgery is:

   A. Diabetes mellitus
   B. Diabetes insipidus
   C. Hyperthyroidism
   D. Adrenal insufficiency

13. The symptoms of a neuroblastoma are determined by:

   A. Nerves that make up tumor
   B. Location of mass
   C. Age of child
   D. Amount of bone marrow suppression

14. Before the initial surgery, parents of a child with a newlydiagnosed Wilms' tumor ask you about their child's prognosis. Your best response is:

   A. "The prognosis cannot be predicted until the tumor is studied."
   B. "The vast majority of children, almost 90%, survive Wilms' tumor."
   C. "With surgery, chemotherapy, and radiation, the prognosis will be excellent."
   D. "The prognosis is usually good, but there are some cases that have poor survival rates."

15. The abdomen of a child with a Wilms' tumor should not be palpated because the pressure could:

   A. Cause extreme pain
   B. Rupture tumor
   C. Disrupt kidney function
   D. Frighten patient

16. Osteosarcoma is often diagnosed when a child:

   A. Fractures leg near tumor
   B. Develops shortened limb
   C. Has x-ray of affected limb for other reasons
   D. Complains of pain and swelling

17. Leukemia occurs when stem cells in the bone marrow produce:

   A. Immature erythrocytes that cannot function
   B. Immature white blood cells that cannot function
   C. Large numbers of platelets
   D. Large numbers of erythrocytes

18. The definitive diagnostic test for leukemia is:

   A. Total platelet count
   B. Lumbar puncture
   C. Bone marrow aspiration
   D. Complete blood cell count

19. Hodgkin's disease is a disorder of:

   A. Lymphatic system
   B. Nervous system
   C. Hematopoietic system
   D. Cardiovascular system

20. The main symptom of Hodgkin's disease is:

   A. Pain in abdomen
   B. Mass in groin
   C. Firm lymphadenopathy
   D. Tenderness in neck

21. The first sign of retinoblastoma is usually:

   A. Cat's-eye reflex
   B. Ptosis
   C. Blurred vision
   D. Blindness

CASE STUDIES

1. Mindy, 2 years old, has a swelling on her left side, below her rib cage. Her mother notices the swelling during Mindy's bath and, concerned, calls the pediatrician the next day to ask about the "lump." Mindy's pediatrician immediately admits the toddler to the hospital, suspecting a Wilms' tumor. After preliminary testing (sonogram and CT scan), surgery is performed to remove the tumor. The tumor is staged at level II.

   Outline the care that Mindy will require from admission through discharge, keeping in mind her developmental stage, and briefly discuss her family's response to the diagnosis.

2. John, 10 years old, is receiving chemotherapy after removal of a neuroblastoma. He is experiencing several unpleasant side effects of the chemotherapy

(nausea and vomiting, anorexia and weight loss, and mouth sores). Describe various medical and nursing interventions that could help manage these side effects.

Suggested Learning Activities

1. Visit a hospital where pediatric cancers are treated. Some areas to investigate are:
   A. Is the hospital actively involved in cancer research?
   B. How are treatment protocols devised?
   C. What support systems are available for parents and families of children being treated?
   D. Are there active family support groups in the area? Are families referred to support groups by the hospital?
   E. Is written information given to parents?

2. Visit a radiation treatment facility. Some areas to investigate include:
   A. How are children oriented to the facility? Do staff hold practice sessions for children before the initial treatment session?
   B. If necessary, how are children restrained?
   C. How are radiation doses and number of treatments determined for children?

3. Contact a local branch of the American Cancer Society. What services does it provide? What information is available for parents about specific childhood cancers? Is there a referral service for families with a member who has cancer?

ANSWERS WITH RATIONALES

Review of Concepts

MATCHING

1.

1. G	2. E	3. H
4. F	5. A	6. D
7. B	8. C	

2.

1. D, E	2. G	3. H
4. A, F	5. B, C	6. I
7. F		

SHORT ESSAY

1. Cancer in adults is often the result of dietary practices, habits, or environmental factors that can be avoided. Thus, prevention of adult cancer is directed at lifestyle changes and interventions. Because children usually develop cancers that are embryonic or oncogenic (genetic) in origin, there are no lifestyle changes that could be instituted to change the incidence of childhood cancer.

2. Many signs and symptoms of cancer are nonspecific; that is, they may also occur in other common childhood illnesses. The five common signs are:
   A. *Pain*—Resulting from neoplasm that directly or indirectly affects nerve receptors.
   B. *Cachexia*—A combination of anorexia, weight loss, anemia, asthenia, and early satiety.
   C. *Anemia*—Resulting from chronic bleeding and iron deficiency.
   D. *Infection*—Resulting from altered or immature immune system.
   E. *Bruising*—Resulting when bone marrow cannot produce enough platelets and bleeding occurs after minor trauma.

3. The three goals of cancer treatment in children are:
   A. *Curative*—Treatment that rids the body of the cancer.
   B. *Supportive*—Treatment that helps the body's defenses (e.g., transfusions, pain management, antibiotics).
   C. *Palliative*—Treatment that makes the child comfortable.

4. Cancer is treated with one or a combination of the following therapies:
   A. Surgery
   B. Chemotherapy
   C. Radiation
   D. Biotherapy
   E. Bone marrow transplantation

5. A protocol is the plan of action for chemotherapy. The type of cancer, its stage, and the particular cell type determine the drug used, dose, and interval of treatment which, in turn, determine the treatment for side effects and needed laboratory studies.

6. Nausea and vomiting may occur immediately or up to 5–6 hours after administration of chemotherapy and may last 48 hours. Nursing interventions may include administering antiemetics if ordered, teaching relaxation techniques, hypnosis, and systematic desensitization to help decrease the symptoms. Encouraging mild exercise and changing the diet to include only easily digested foods in the 12 hours before therapy may also be helpful.

7. The goal of bone marrow transplantation is to give a lethal dose of therapy to kill the cancer, and then resupply the body with bone marrow stem cells, either from the child's own marrow previously removed and stored or from a compatible donor.

8. When the family is in the initial phase of shock, they will not retain much information. However, this is a time when large amounts of information must be presented and many decisions made. Continual restatement and clarification of the information is a responsibility of the health care team. Providing written information enables the parents to retain more of the content and refer to it later.

   Parents need opportunities to ask questions and express their concerns and feelings about the diagnosis. Techniques such as reflecting, restating, and observing nonverbal behaviors will help to facilitate this communication process. Many parents fear telling the child and siblings about the diagnosis, as well as telling people outside the immediate family. Family conferences with the health care team enable all members to express feelings and learn about care and treatment together.

   The role of the parents in their child's care must be emphasized. They are very important in maintaining their child's well-being, and they need to be supported in that role throughout their child's treatment. The family will encounter tremendous stressors, and referral to social service agencies and family counseling may be welcomed.

9. The three common treatment-induced threats to body image are hair loss, surgical scars, and cushingoid changes. Hair loss occurs when the head is shaved for cranial surgery or when hair falls out during chemotherapy. This is particularly devasting to adolescents, because physical appearance is very important to them. They fear ridicule and rejection by their peer group. Surgical scars or changes that are obvious and not easily concealed are also very upsetting. Cushingoid changes, which occur with the use of corticosteroids, include the development of a round and flushed face, prominent cheeks, double chin, and generalized obesity. The obesity also causes stretch marks that are often permanent even after the weight is lost.

10. Support systems outside of the immediate family include the extended family, friends, governmental agencies, insurance coverage, religious affiliations, cultural support systems, and the school system. Families need to be encouraged to identify supports that are available to them and to use them.

11. Both students and teachers benefit from preparation for a child's return to school after cancer treatment. Discuss and role play how the child can tell friends about physical changes from the cancer treatment. A nurse or child life specialist can visit the child's class to explain what the child is experiencing and meet with teacher to devise a plan for preparing classmates.

12. Complications of treatment for brain tumors are significant. They include severe infections, seizure activity, sensorimotor defects, hydrocephalus, growth problems, endocrine problems (such as hypothyroidism), decrease in intelligence quotient (IQ), frank mental retardation, memory deficits, and selective attention deficits.

13. The malignant white blood cells rapidly fill the bone marrow, replacing stem cells that produce erythrocytes and other blood cell components, such as platelets. This decreases the circulating levels of these cells. Abnormal bleeding occurs because of the reduced number of platelets.

Critical Thinking: Application/Analysis

MULTIPLE CHOICE

1. C. The effectiveness of chemotherapy is determined in part by the rate of cell replication. Cells are more vulnerable to destruction during the process of division. Because many cancerous cells multiply at a rate more rapid than that of normal cells, more of these cells would be undergoing division at any given time and, hence, would be damaged or destroyed.

2. B. Anabolic androgenic steroids are carcinogens, chemicals that, when combined with genetic traits and other carcinogens, can cause cancer.

3. B. The mucosal tissues that line the gastrointestinal tract normally divide very rapidly because they are constantly being sloughed and replaced. Because they are rapidly dividing, they are more sensitive to chemotherapy drugs. It is common

for children to have sores in their mouths and diarrhea when they are undergoing chemotherapy.

4. D. The child must be placed in the same position for each radiation treatment. The child must lie completely still for the entire session, which can last 10 to 20 minutes. Very young and anxious children may need to be sedated for these treatments.

5. B. Thrombocytopenia, a decrease in the number of platelets, can result in spontaneous bleeding into the tissues from the blood vessels. Prevention of bruises will decrease the risk of bleeding.

6. C. When the immune system is suppressed, the child is vulnerable to any infection, which can progress to septic shock or death.

7. A. The implanted device is under the child's skin. The child can go swimming, because there is no point of entry to become contaminated. Such activity is not possible with nonimplanted devices.

8. C. Children who are undergoing chemotherapy often experience side effects, such as taste changes, mouth sores, and nausea, that can decrease nutritional intake. They will be more willing to eat foods that are familiar (e.g., favorite foods).

9. A. Handwashing kills organisms and is the most effective measure in preventing infection.

10. B. Cerebral capillaries regulate the rate at which substances in the blood permeate brain tissue. Because some chemotherapy drugs enter brain tissue very slowly, the concentration of the drug is very low in the area of the tumor and therefore not very effective.

11. B. Vomiting is a nonspecific sign of a brain tumor caused by increased intracranial pressure.

12. B. Removal of tumors in the midline of the brain can result in damage to the pituitary gland, which secretes the antidiuretic hormone vasopressin. This results in diabetes insipidus. Polyuria and polydipsia, if untreated, can lead to dehydration and hypotension. This condition is managed by replacement of vasopressin (see Chapter 20).

13. B. A neuroblastoma is a small, hard, nontender mass. Symptoms depend on where the mass is located (e.g., dyspnea occurs if the tumor is located in the mediastinum).

14. A. Prognosis is determined by tumor staging and histologic finding. Therefore, before surgery it is impossible to discuss prognosis with the family without giving vague information.

15. B. In its early stages Wilms' tumor is confined to the kidney and therefore encapsulated. The chances of survival are much greater if the tumor is not ruptured before or during surgery. If it ruptures, the tumor cells may be seeded throughout the abdomen.

16. D. Initial symptoms of osteosarcoma are pain and swelling in the bone.

17. B. The white blood cells produced do not function normally. They proliferate quickly, filling the bone marrow and eventually replacing the normal white blood cells. As the normal white blood cells are replaced, cellular and humoral immunity are reduced, leaving the body vulnerable to infections.

18. C. The bone marrow aspiration reveals immature and abnormal lymphoblasts and hypercellular marrow; this is a differential test.

19. A. Hodgkin's disease occurs in the lymph nodes, part of the lymphatic system.

20. C. The main symptom of Hodgkin's disease is a nontender, firm lymphadenopathy. Other symptoms that can occur are fever, night sweats, and weight loss.

21. A. Retinoblastoma, an interocular malignancy of the retina, is usually first noted as a white reflection in the pupil (termed cat's-eye reflex). Normally a red reflex is seen when light is shown on the retina. This may be seen in family pictures in which everyone has "red eyes" except the affected toddler, who has only one "red eye."

CASE STUDIES

1. At 2 years of age, Mindy is struggling with autonomy and the need to feel secure. Admission to the hospital interferes with most attempts at autonomy. The admission is very fast, and Mindy's parents are upset and unprepared. They may be unable to give Mindy the attention she needs to help her feel secure. Before and after surgery, it is best if her parents can remain with her most of the time, soothing and distracting her from stressful procedures and events. This will require the activation of family support systems, such as home care for siblings, time off from work, etc.

   Mindy will require normal postoperative care (respiratory care, pain control, infection surveillance, etc.). See Chapter 4 for additional information on pediatric surgery. Special attention needs to be focused on fluid monitoring, because Mindy has only one kidney remaining. Hypovolemia and third-space fluid shifts, as well as shock, are also possible. Before discharge a central line will probably be inserted for chemotherapy, and Mindy's parents need instruction in care and maintenance of this line.

   Mindy's parents will be experiencing shock because of the suddenness of her diagnosis and admission. There is no delay between diagnosis and surgery because of the danger that the tumor may rupture. Her parents thus have little time to come to terms with the diagnosis. They will receive much information and make many decisions within a very short time. The health care team needs to anticipate the retention of only a small fraction of this information by the parents and the need to reteach information as necessary. Mindy's parents will have many questions about her prognosis and future treatment that cannot be answered until after surgery, and this can be very frustrating to them. After surgery, family–health team conferences will be held to answer as many questions as possible. An assessment of support systems available to the family is important, so that appropriate referrals can be made.

   Anticipatory guidance before discharge focuses on upcoming medical treatment (e.g., chemotherapy) and the side effects that Mindy will experience. Mindy's parents need to understand how they can help their child before chemotherapy begins and during treatment. They should be encouraged to maintain a normal environment at home. Growth and development should be promoted with age-appropriate toys, and Mindy should be encouraged to participate in normal play activities. Therapeutic play activities that can be used at home to decrease Mindy's anxiety can be discussed with her parents. Mindy's parents will also need education about promoting nutritional intake, signs of infection, preventing infection (particularly during periods of neutropenia from chemotherapy), administering medications at home, medication side effects, and methods of controlling pain. Referrals should be made to a home care agency, cancer support groups, and the American Cancer Society for additional information and resources.

2. At 10 years of age John fears loss of function and altered body image. His experience with chemo-

therapy has been distressing because he is not in control and his body image is changing because of his weight loss. Interventions that would help manage these side effects include:

A. *Nausea and vomiting*—Use of antiemetics may be helpful. Other nonpharmacological measures include relaxation techniques, hypnosis, and systematic desensitization (hypnotic process that progressively reduces reaction to a medication that causes a strong emotional or physical response). Other interventions include mild exercise and change of diet (e.g., eating only easily digested foods 12 hours before chemotherapy).

B. *Anorexia and weight loss*—Identify any changes in taste that have occurred and encourage preferred food choices. Consult with a dietitian to modify John's diet. If dietary modifications are unsuccessful, hyperalimentation may be necessary.

C. *Mouth sores*—These are a large factor in John's reluctance to eat. Encourage good oral hygiene, using a soft foam wand instead of a tooth brush, which can damage the mucosa. Avoid using commercial mouthwashes, which contain alcohol that increases drying of the mouth. Using an antifungal agent will reduce the possibility of candidal infection.

15

ALTERATIONS IN GASTROINTESTINAL FUNCTION

Chapter Overview

Chapter 15 focuses on some of the common gastrointestinal (GI) disorders that affect children. Structural defects, hernias, inflammatory disorders, and ostomies are discussed. Disorders of motility, intestinal parasitic disorders, feeding disorders, malabsorption disorders, hepatic disorders, and injuries to the GI system are also presented.

Learning Objectives

After studying this chapter, you should be able to:
*   Identify significant differences between the adult and pediatric GI systems.
*   Compare and contrast the structural defects that cause dysfunction in the GI system.
*   Describe the nursing management of children with cleft lip and/or palate defects.
*   Formulate discharge instructions for children following cleft lip repair.
*   Describe the clinical manifestations of various structural disorders that cause GI obstruction and the medical and nursing management of children with these disorders.
*   Describe the care of children with diaphragmatic or umbilical hernias.
*   Discuss the nursing assessment and management of children with inflammatory disorders of the GI system.
*   Discuss the impact of an ostomy on the growth

and development of an adolescent.
*   Describe the nursing management of children with motility disorders.
*   Describe the transmission and clinical manifestations of common intestinal parasites.
*   Describe the anticipatory guidance needed for children with feeding and malabsorptive disorders.
*   Discuss the nursing assessment and management of children with hepatic disorders.
*   Recognize the effects of common toxic agents and describe the treatment of children poisoned by these agents.
*   Discuss common abdominal injuries that can occur in children.

Review of Concepts

MATCHING

Match the items in list 1 with the appropriate word or phrase in list 2. (*Note:* Items may be used more than once.)

1. Abdominal Obstructive Disorders

LIST 1
A. Pyloric stenosis
B. Intussusception
C. Rectal agenesis
D. Esophageal atresia
E. Hirschsprung's disease

LIST 2

1. ____ Failure to pass meconium
2. ____ Choking and emesis with first feeding after birth
3. ____ Olive-shaped mass in right upper quadrant of abdomen
4. ____ Sausage-shaped mass in right upper quadrant of abdomen
5. ____ Projectile vomiting
6. ____ Nonbilious vomitus
7. ____ Currant jellylike stools
8. ____ Excessive salivation and drooling
9. ____ Acute abdominal pain
10. ____ Ribbonlike stools

2. Intestinal Parasitic Infections

LIST 1
A. Giardiasis
B. Enterobiasis (pinworm)
C. Ascariasis (roundworm)
D. Hookworm disease

LIST 2
1. ____ Intense perianal itching
2. ____ Larvae can migrate from intestines to lungs
3. ____ Larvae attach to and penetrate skin, then enter bloodstream
4. ____ Eggs are excreted in stool
5. ____ Transmitted through unfiltered water
6. ____ Eggs are laid near anal opening
7. ____ Watery stools
8. ____ Transmitted through direct contact with infected soil containing larvae

3. Commonly Ingested Toxic Agents

LIST 1
A. Oven cleaner
B. Kerosene
C. Acetaminophen
D. Iron
E. Salicylate

LIST 2
1. ____ Induce vomiting
2. ____ Child at risk for airway obstruction
3. ____ Severe burning of mouth
4. ____ Do not induce vomiting
5. ____ Bloody stools
6. ____ Child at risk for pneumonia
7. ____ Tinnitus
8. ____ Pain in right upper quadrant of abdomen
9. ____ Metabolic acidosis
10. ____ Lethargy

SHORT ESSAY

1. Outline a discharge plan for an infant who has undergone repair of a cleft lip defect.

2. A 14-year-old child has swallowed a bottle of acetaminophen tablets. Describe the implications of this act, and outline the treatment of this patient.

3. You are discussing accidental poisoning with the parents of a 1-year-old infant. Describe the anticipatory guidance you would give this family.

Critical Thinking: Application/Analysis

MULTIPLE CHOICE

Select the best answer.

1. Infants often experience abdominal distention because they:

    A. Are not burped adequately during feedings
    B. Swallow air during and between feedings
    C. Have a deficiency of digestive enzymes
    D. Are given cow's milk instead of formula

2. To decrease their risk of having children with orofacial clefts, women who are planning a pregnancy are advised to:

    A. Take extra vitamin C
    B. Increase their iron intake
    C. Avoid use of alcohol
    D. Take folic acid supplements

3. Repair of a cleft lip is often begun in early infancy:

   A. To facilitate speech development
   B. To prevent development of infections
   C. For cosmetic reasons
   D. To facilitate normal dentition

4. Following a cleft palate repair, parents need to be cautioned to:

   A. Refrain from looking in infant's mouth
   B. Give only liquids until healing is complete
   C. Avoid using metal spoons or straws
   D. Offer a pacifier to soothe infant

5. During the initial feeding, a newborn begins to choke and return fluid from the mouth and nose. The nurse would:

   A. Resume feeding as soon as infant has recovered from choking spell
   B. Immediately stop feeding infant
   C. Allow infant to rest, then try again
   D. Keep infant NPO for 12 hours, then give another feeding

6. The vomitus of an infant with pyloric stenosis does not contain bile because:

   A. Bile duct has become obstructed
   B. Bile is not produced until child is older
   C. Vomiting occurs too quickly
   D. Obstruction is located above bile duct

7. Before initiating a gastrostomy feeding, the residual in the stomach from the previous feeding is measured and:

   A. Discarded
   B. Returned to stomach
   C. Replaced with fresh formula
   D. Diluted with water and returned to stomach

8. An infant with pyloric stenosis is at risk for developing:

   A. Metabolic acidosis
   B. Metabolic alkalosis
   C. Respiratory acidosis
   D. Respiratory alkalosis

9. Diagnosis of gastroesophageal reflux is confirmed by:

   A. One episode of aspiration pneumonia
   B. Esophageal pH probe monitoring
   C. MRI of the abdomen and chest
   D. Number and severity of vomiting episodes

10. Infants with gastroesophageal reflux should be positioned:

    A. Supine or on side
    B. In an infant seat with head up
    C. Prone with head elevated
    D. Prone with head lower than feet

11. Education for parents of an infant with an umbilical hernia would include which of the following statements?

    A. "Place a wide band over the hernia to keep it flat."
    B. "Notify your doctor if the hernia does not close by 12 months of age."
    C. "Surgical closure is performed at around 18 months of age."
    D. "Notify your doctor if you cannot push the bowel back into the abdomen."

12. To prevent impaction of a child with mild Hirschsprung's disease, management includes stool softeners and:

    A. Isotonic saline enemas
    B. Daily laxatives
    C. Oil retention enemas
    D. Soap suds enemas

13. Abdominal assessment of a child with appendicitis often reveals:

    A. Constant pain in left lower abdomen
    B. Rebound tenderness following palpation
    C. Abdominal distention with no bowel sounds
    D. Visible peristaltic waves over abdomen

14. A major concern of an adolescent following abdominal surgery is:

    A. Appearance of incision after healing
    B. Side effects of prescribed medications
    C. Prevention of other complications
    D. Visits from family and friends

15. An infant with a diaphragmatic hernia is positioned:

    A. Flat on abdomen
    B. With head and chest elevated
    C. With head and chest lowered
    D. On right side

16. A recently ruptured appendix is suspected when:

    A. Abdominal pain shifts from left side to right side
    B. Temperature drops below normal
    C. Abdominal pain is suddenly relieved
    D. Vomiting and diarrhea intensify

17. A nursing priority when caring for a child following abdominal surgery is to:

    A. Give narcotic analgesics every 2 to 3 hours
    B. Maintain child on bed rest
    C. Have child turn, cough, and deep breathe every hour
    D. Force fluids by mouth

18. Parent education is especially important before testing for a Meckel's diverticulum because:

    A. Testing is painful
    B. Abdomen must be relaxed
    C. All barium must be expelled from bowel
    D. Radioactive material is used in scanning

19. Children with gastroenteritis often receive intravenous (IV) fluids to correct dehydration. How would you explain the need for IV fluids to a 3-year-old child?

    A. "The doctor wants you to get more water, and this is the best way to get it."
    B. "Your stomach is sick and won't let you drink anything. The water going through the tube will help you feel better."
    C. "See how much better your roommate is feeling with his IV? You will get better, too."
    D. "The water in the IV goes into your veins and replaces the water you have lost from vomiting and diarrhea."

20. Which of the following foods would be appropriate for a child recovering from gastroenteritis?

    A. Yogurt
    B. Cheese
    C. Ginger ale
    D. Toast

21. The best strategy to prevent constipation in a child is to:

    A. Give bananas and yogurt for snacks
    B. Give stool softeners daily
    C. Place child on toilet twice a day
    D. Give fresh fruit and juices for snacks

22. Parents of an infant with colic are often exhausted and frustrated because:

    A. Infant is hungry all the time
    B. They fear infant is malnourished
    C. They do not know what formula to use
    D. Attempts to quiet infant are ineffective

23. A common food that may cause a sensitivivy reaction is:

    A. Rice
    B. Cow's milk
    C. Applesauce
    D. Beef

24. Which of the following foods would be appropriate for a child with celiac disease?

    A. Eggs and toast
    B. Cornbread and baked beans
    C. Oatmeal and milk
    D. Beef and gravy

25. Infants with biliary atresia become very irritable as the disease progresses because of:

   A. Abdominal distention
   B. Difficulty breathing
   C. Abdominal pain
   D. Intense itching

26. The spread of hepatitis A can be prevented by:

   A. Proper handwashing and disposal of diapers
   B. Immunization with hepatitis B vaccine
   C. Protected sexual intercourse
   D. Avoiding parenteral drug use

27. Medical personnel can protect themselves from infection with hepatitis B by:

   A. Careful handwashing
   B. Immunization with hepatitis B vaccine
   C. Avoiding accidental needle sticks
   D. Isolating patients with hepatitis

28. A child complaining of abdominal pain after a fall from a bicycle should be assessed for:

   A. Ruptured stomach
   B. Bruised intestine
   C. Fractured rib
   D. Ruptured spleen

29. Vomiting is not induced following ingestion of hydrocarbons to prevent:

   A. Pharyngeal swelling
   B. Burning of esophagus
   C. Aspiration pneumonia
   D. Hemoptysis

30. Which statement by a parent would cause you to investigate the potential for lead poisoning in the family?

   A. "We just refinished all of our woodwork."
   B. "Our furnace is brand new."
   C. "We have replaced all the ceilings in the house."
   D. "Our brick house is 20 years old."

CASE STUDIES

1. The birth of an infant with a cleft lip and/or palate defect can be devastating to new parents. Describe how you would approach these parents, and outline a teaching plan for this family.

2. Describe the developmental impact that a colostomy would have on a 16-year-old adolescent, and discuss various strategies to enhance coping and promote growth in the adolescent. (*Hint:* It may be helpful to review the information presented in Chapter 2.)

Suggested Learning Activities

1. Examine your home for substances that could be poisonous to a young child (e.g., medications, cleaning supplies, plants). How could you make your home safer for a child?

2. Many children with biliary atresia will eventually need a liver transplant. Every hospital has an organ procurement policy and procedure. Interview a nurse who is involved with organ procurement at your local hospital. Some possible questions and issues to explore are:
   A. How is the decision reached to donate organs?
   B. Which organ banks are notified?
   C. How is the organ harvest actually performed?

ANSWERS WITH RATIONALES

Review of Concepts

MATCHING

1.

1. C, E	2. D	3. A
4. B	5. A	6. A
7. B	8. D	9. B
10. E		

2.

1. B	2. C	3. D
4. C, D	5. A	6. B
7. A	8. D	

3.

1. C, D, E	2. A	3. A
4. A, B	5. D	6. B
7. E	8. C	9. D, E
10. B		

SHORT ESSAY

1. Care at home would include:
   A. Monitoring suture lines for signs of infection
   B. Cleaning sutures and mouth after feeding
   C. Positioning infant on side or back only
   D. Use of elbow restraint until lip is healed (removing restraint and exercising arms every 2 hours)
   E. Medicating for pain as needed
   F. Use of Asepto syringe or dropper to feed infant and avoiding use of a pacifier until lip is healed or until approved by physician

2. Many troubled teens make suicide gestures out of anger or in an attempt to manipulate others. They often use acetaminophen because they do not consider this drug to be dangerous. In large doses, however, acetaminophen can cause damage to the liver and even death. When the ingestion is discovered, vomiting is induced immediately to rid the body of any drug still in the stomach. Blood levels are assessed, and the amount of antidote (Mucomyst or NAC) needed is calculated. Mucomyst is given orally for several days. The prognosis may be uncertain for several days or weeks.

3. Anticipatory guidance about accidental poisoning would include:
   A. Normal growth and development, emphasizing infant's tendency to place everything in the mouth and increased abilities in mobility and reaching
   B. Proper storage of cleansers, medications, and other potential poisons in locked cabinets and use of warning stickers (e.g., Mr. Yuk)
   C. Use of childproof caps
   D. Storage of poisonous materials in original containers, not in food or beverage containers (e.g., soda bottle)
   E. Removing all house plants from infant's play area
   F. Using caution when visiting areas that are not childproofed
   G. Keeping two bottles of ipecac syrup per child in the house

Critical Thinking: Application/Analysis

MULTIPLE CHOICE

1. C. Infants have a deficiency of amylase, lipase, and trypsin until about 4 to 6 months of age. Incomplete digestion causes gas and flatus, resulting in abdominal distention.

2. D. Folic acid supplementation during pregnancy has been shown to decrease the incidence of

neural tube defects by 25%–50%. Because these defects occur during the first trimester, it is more beneficial to be taking folic acid around the time of conception.

3. A. Closure of the cleft lip enables the infant to form a seal around the nipple, which facilitates sucking. Sucking motions strengthen the muscles that will be used later for speech.

4. C. Any hard object placed in the mouth can disrupt the suture line.

5. B. These are symptoms of a tracheoesophageal fistula; continued feeding could lead to aspiration pneumonia.

6. D. For bile to be present in the vomitus, it must enter the stomach from the duodenum. In pyloric stenosis, the intestine is compressed at the outlet of the stomach. Therefore the bile cannot enter the stomach.

7. B. Discarding the residual formula could lead to electrolyte imbalance because acid from the stomach also would be discarded.

8. B. The infant is losing excessive amounts of acid from the stomach with each episode of vomiting, leading to metabolic alkalosis.

9. B. One way to confirm gastroesophageal reflux is to insert a small catheter through the nose and into the esophagus and leave it in place for 18–24 hours to measure the pH over a period of time. When the child is in various positions and eating certain foods and drinks, the probe will show the reflux of the acidic stomach contents into the normally nonacidic esophagus.

10. C. Placing the infant in the prone position with the head up helps to prevent aspiration if reflux should occur.

11. D. Strangulation of the bowel occurs if the bowel becomes caught in the fibrous umbilical ring, causing obstruction. This is a medical emergency.

12. A. Peristalsis of the normal bowel can move stool through a small portion of a ganglionic colon; however, the stool needs to be soft. When constipation does occur, using isotonic saline to irrigate the bowel facilitates the removal of the firmer stool. Saline is used to prevent excess absorption of free water through the bowel into the general circulation, preventing water intoxication.

13. B. When the right lower quadrant is palpated, the pain becomes worse when the examiner's hand is withdrawn.

14. A. Adolescents are very concerned about the surgical scar because they are preoccupied with their body image.

15. B. Elevating the head and chest facilitates the downward movement of the abdominal contents, which would otherwise protrude through the hole in the diaphragm into the thorax, causing severe respiratory distress.

16. C. Rupture of the appendix immediately relieves the pain resulting from the pressure within the appendix. However, this relief is only temporary. As peritoneal infection develops, the pain returns.

17. C. The child is unwilling to cough because of the incisional pain and takes only short breaths, which can lead to atelectasis and pneumonia. Splinting the abdominal incision with a pillow, rolled blanket, or towel decreases the child's pain when coughing and deep breathing.

18. D. Many people are afraid of exposure to radioactivity. Parents must be given information about the material being used and the length of time it will remain in the body. They also need to know how it will be excreted from the body and how to dispose of it appropriately.

19. B. By age 3, a child uses words as symbols and has a rudimentary understanding of cause-and-effect relationships. Children in this age group are egocentric, so they are unable to see things

from another person's perspective. It is important to explain procedures and equipment in simple terms that relate directly to the child.

20. D. Once dehydration is corrected, a CRAM diet can be started if tolerated. The CRAM diet contains complex carbohydrates (cereals, toast, pasta), rice, and milk.

21. D. A high-fiber diet with increased fluids is the best method to promote regular bowel movements in children.

22. D. Infants with colic cry loudly and continuously, often for hours. They do not respond to normal cuddling behavior because of the pain they are experiencing. Parents become frustrated when they are unable to calm the frantic, crying infant and begin to fear that the infant is very ill.

23. B. Cow's milk proteins can cause a GI response of diarrhea, vomiting, and abdominal pain. In infants the diarrhea is often watery, blood-streaked, and mucoid.

24. B. Children with celiac disease can eat rice and corn, which do not contain the protein gluten. Care must be taken to read labels of all prepared foods, since most flour used in food preparation is made from wheat, barley, rye, or oats, all of which contain gluten. Wheat flour is also a common ingredient in sauces and gravies. Children with celiac disease should eat only sauces or gravies thickened with cornstarch.

25. D. Biliary atresia causes altered bile flow from the liver to the duodenum, resulting in inflammation and fibrotic changes in the liver. Accumulation of bilirubin leads to jaundice, which results in severe pruritis.

26. A. Hepatitis A is spread by the fecal–oral route. Washing hands before and after toileting and disposing of soiled diapers can prevent the spread of this disease.

27. B. Hepatitis B immunization is recommended for all health care workers and others at risk for exposure to hepatitis B.

28. D. The spleen is a solid organ located under the left rib cage margin. The handlebars of a bicycle can strike the child in the upper abdomen during a fall, causing blunt trauma to the spleen. Because the spleen is solid and highly vascular, rupture can result in severe hemorrhage.

29. C. Aspiration of hydrocarbons, such as gasoline and paint thinners, place children at high risk for severe pneumonia.

30. A. Many parents do not realize that when they remove paint from the woodwork in their home by sanding, they release large quantities of paint dust into the air. This dust settles throughout the home. If the paint contains lead, large doses of lead may be inhaled and ingested by all members of the family. The children are at greater risk of permanent damage because they retain more lead in their bodies than adults do.

CASE STUDIES

1. Encourage the parents to hold and cuddle their infant, focusing on the entire infant, not just on the cleft lip or palate. Discuss the usual sequence of events for surgical correction and show them "before" and "after" pictures of a child who has had this type of correction. Anticipate feeding difficulties and work with the parents to find the best method to feed their infant. Anticipatory guidance would include instructing parents that the infant will need follow-up care, including plastic surgery, hearing assessments, and orthodontia. Parents should be advised that ear infections are common and speech therapy is often necessary for children with cleft lip or palate.

2. In the identity vs. role confusion stage (Erikson), the adolescent searches for self-identify, moving away from the parents and relying more on peers. However, the adolescent with a colostomy may fear ridicule or shunning if the peer group finds out about the colostomy and thus may withdraw from peers and become more dependent on the parents instead. A colostomy is also a tremendous insult to one's body image, which is a part of self-identity. In the genital stage (Freud) the adolescent focuses on genital function and relationships. However, adolescents with a colostomy may be reluctant to pursue a close relationship, fearing rejection. In the formal operations stage (Piaget), the adolescent is capable of mature, abstract thought. However, educational instruction often is given to the parents rather than to the adolescent.

Strategies to enhance coping and growth would include introducing the adolescent to another teen who has a colostomy or has had one in the past. Such a relationship can provide the adolescent with a peer with whom to discuss his or her most pressing concerns. Independence is enhanced by directing all education to the adolescent rather than to the parents. Following surgery, the adolescent should be encouraged to handle all colostomy equipment and appliances since practice will enhance the adolescent's feelings of competence. Referral to an adolescent support group can provide an outlet for expression of feelings as well as peer relationships that help promote independence.

16

ALTERATIONS IN GENITOURINARY FUNCTION

Chapter Overview

Chapter 16 focuses on the care of children with alterations in genitourinary function. Pediatric differences in the genitourinary system are presented, followed by a discussion of selected structural defects of the urinary system. Next, urinary tract infections, enuresis, renal disorders, structural defects of the reproductive system, and sexually transmitted diseases are discussed, with emphasis on medical and nursing management of each disorder.

Learning Objectives

After studying this chapter, you should be able to:
- Identify the differences between the adult and pediatric genitourinary systems.
- Describe selected structural defects of the urinary and reproductive systems and the medical and nursing management of children with these defects.
- Identify the cause of most urinary tract infections.
- Discuss the treatment of urinary tract infections and describe an educational plan to prevent future infections in children of various ages.
- Describe enuresis and the medical and nursing management of children with this disorder.

- Explain the etiology of selected renal disorders and the medical and nursing management of children with these disorders.
- Differentiate between hemodialysis and peritoneal dialysis.
- Differentiate among selected sexually transmitted diseases.
- Describe the educational plan for an adolescent diagnosed with a sexually transmitted disease.

Review of Concepts

MATCHING

Match the items in list 1 with the appropriate word or phrase in list 2. (*Note:* Items may be used more than once.)

1. Clinical Manifestations of Common Renal Disorders

LIST 1
A. Minimal change nephrotic syndrome
B. Acute renal failure
C. Hemolytic-uremic syndrome
D. Acute postinfectious glomerulonephritis

LIST 2
1. ____ Tea-colored urine
2. ____ Petechiae
3. ____ Edema
4. ____ Nausea and vomiting
5. ____ Abdominal pain

2. Clinical Manifestations of Sexually Transmitted Diseases

LIST 1
A. Chlamydia
B. Genital herpes
C. Gonorrhea
D. Syphilis

LIST 2
1. ____ Dysuria in males
2. ____ Painless lesion (chancre) in both sexes
3. ____ Purulent vaginal discharge, cervicitis
4. ____ Painful or itchy ulcers in perianal area
5. ____ Pelvic inflammatory disease
6. ____ Yellow urethral discharge in males
7. ____ Diffuse rash, malaise, fever
8. ____ Enlarged lymph nodes near lesions

SHORT ESSAY

1. Describe vesicoureteral reflux and explain its role in urinary tract infections.

2. Describe measures that are effective in preventing urinary tract infections.

3. Describe six treatment approaches for enuresis.

4. List ways to monitor edema in a child with minimal change nephrotic syndrome (MCNS).

5. Compare hemodialysis with peritoneal dialysis.

6. Describe signs of peritonitis that may occur in children receiving peritoneal dialysis.

7. Children with acute postinfectious glomerulonephritis (APIGN) often are anorexic. Give several suggestions for strategies to meet an anorexic child's daily nutritional requirements.

8. Many children receive corticosteroids for renal disorders. What information should be given to the child and/or parents at the beginning of steroid therapy?

Critical Thinking: Application/Analysis

MULTIPLE CHOICE

Select the best answer.

1. Bladder training of children less than 2 years of age is usually unsuccessful because:

   A. Bladder capacity is still small
   B. They cannot understand the concept
   C. Nerve development is insufficient
   D. They are usually not interested

2. In bladder exstrophy the infant's skin must be protected from:

   A. Leaking urine
   B. Oozing stool
   C. Pressure sores
   D. Draining blood

3. An infant with hypospadias is not circumcised because:

   A. Scar formation could jeopardize repair of defect
   B. Defect often extends through foreskin
   C. Foreskin tissue is absent
   D. Foreskin tissue will be used to repair defect

4. Hydropnephrosis is commonly caused by:

   A. Ureteral obstruction
   B. Trauma
   C. Dehydration
   D. Drug toxicity

5. Most urinary tract infections in young girls are attributed to:

A. Small bladder size
B. Bladder neck obstruction
C. Short urethra
D. Poor fluid intake

6. Which of the following fluids can help to prevent urinary tract infections?

A. Apple juice
B. Water
C. Orange juice
D. Cranberry juice

7. Nocturnal enuresis occurs with high frequency in children:

A. With history of depression
B. Whose parents have history of enuresis
C. Whose parents are strict disciplinarians
D. Who also have diurnal enuresis

8. The primary laboratory indicator for minimal change nephrotic syndrome (MCNS) is:

A. Glucosuria
B. Massive proteinuria
C. Hyperglycemia
D. Hyperalbuminemia

9. To reduce massive edema in MCNS, the physician may order:

A. IV albumin
B. Antibiotics
C. IV normal saline
D. Potassium

10. The child with MCNS should follow a diet:

A. Low in protein
B. Without added salt
C. High in calories
D. Low in calories

11. Most clinical manifestations of renal failure can be attributed to:

A. Electrolyte imbalances
B. Dehydration
C. Infection
D. Bleeding

12. A medication commonly used to treat hyperkalemia is:

A. Erythropoietin
B. Sodium chloride
C. Kayexalate
D. Spironolactone

13. The child undergoing hemodialysis needs to be monitored carefully for:

A. Thirst
B. Hypersensitivity
C. Fluid balance
D. Hunger

14. The child with acute renal failure is extremely susceptible to nosocomial infections as a result of:

A. Leukopenia
B. Nephrotoxicity of antibiotics
C. Inability of kidney to filter bacteria
D. Numerous invasive procedures

15. Dietary management in chronic renal failure is focused on limiting demand on the kidneys and:

A. Maximizing caloric intake
B. Limiting calcium intake
C. Preventing diarrhea and constipation
D. Maximizing sodium and potassium intake

16. Because of the reduced glomerular filtration rate in renal failure:

A. Medications excreted by kidneys are withheld
B. Medication dosages must be adjusted
C. Vitamins are withheld
D. Salt in diet is encouraged

17. An early symptom of acute postinfectious glomerulonephritis (APIGN) is:

A. Massive proteinuria
B. Hematuria
C. Hypotension
D. Leukocytosis

18. Failure of a testis to descend from the abdomen into the scrotum will result in:

    A. Abscess formation
    B. Sterility of that testis
    C. Bowel obstruction
    D. Hypertrophy of other testis

19. The postoperative priority following orchiopexy is:

    A. Providing wound care
    B. Monitoring fluid balance
    C. Monitoring priapism
    D. Providing prosthetic care

20. Initial diagnosis of a hydrocele is usually confirmed by means of:

    A. CT scanning
    B. Ultrasonography
    C. Transillumination
    D. Percussion

21. An infant with a large hydrocele should be assessed often for:

    A. Descended testis
    B. Incarcerated hernia
    C. Bruising
    D. Adequate urinary output

CASE STUDIES

1. Yolanda, 14 years old, is admitted to the hospital with high fever, dysuria, frequency, and pain in her left flank. She is diagnosed with pyelonephritis. A culture of her urine yields *Escherichia coli*. Outline an appropriate education plan for Yolanda and her parents.

2. Michael, 15 years old, contacts his physician because he is having a yellow, puslike urethral discharge, frequency, and pain on urination. A culture of the discharge is positive for gonorrhea. Describe the treatment Michael will receive and outline a patient education plan for this sexually transmitted disease.

Suggested Learning Activities

1. Contact a dialysis unit in your area regarding use of dialysis for pediatric patients.
   A. Are any children being treated in the unit?
   B. How well do children comply with their therapeutic regimens?
   C. What measures are taken to keep the children occupied during a treatment?

2. Visit a hospital that performs kidney transplants. Some areas to investigate include:
   A. What is the most common reason for a kidney transplant?
   B. How are the donor kidneys obtained?
   C. How long do children usually wait for a kidney?
   D. What medical regimen is followed after transplantation to prevent rejection of the kidney?

ANSWERS WITH RATIONALES

Review of Concepts

MATCHING

1.
1. D	2. C	3. A, B, D
4. A, B	5. A, D	

2.
1. A, C	2. D	3. A, C
4. B	5. A, C	6. A, C
7. D	8. B	

SHORT ESSAY

1. Urine normally flows from the kidneys through the ureters in one direction only and enters the bladder at the ureterostoma. During micturition (voiding) the bladder contracts and the urethral sphincters relax, allowing the urine to flow easily out of the bladder. The bladder normally empties completely with only minimal residual urine remaining.

   Reflux occurs when urine flows up the ureters during micturition. After the bladder empties, the urine flows back into the bladder, providing a reservoir for bacteria. A voiding cystourethrogram (VCUG) is used to identify the presence of obstructions, reflux, and residual urine. In this test a contrast medium is instilled in the blader via a catheter. The catheter is then removed and the bladder, ureters, and urethra are visualized during micturition.

2. To prevent urinary tract infections, it is recommended that children avoid taking bubble baths and using hot tubs, wear cotton underwear, avoid tight-fitting pants, wipe the perineum from front to back after voiding and bowel movements, and avoid "holding" urine by urinating more often during the day. Girls who are sexually active should be instructed to void before and after sexual intercourse.

3. Common approaches for treating enuresis are:
   A. *Fluid restriction*—Fluid is limited after the dinner meal.
   B. *Bladder exercises*—The child drinks a large amount and then holds urine as long as possible. Exercises should continue for 6 months.
   C. *Timed voiding*—Child voids every 2 hours to train the bladder to empty completely and avoid overdistension.
   D. *Enuresis alarms*—A detector strip that is attached to the child's pants. When wetting occurs, the alarm sounds a buzzer to allow the child to awaken and get up and finish voiding in the bathroom.
   E. *Reward system*—Realistic goals are set for the child, and dry days or nights are reinforced with stars and stickers on a chart.
   F. *Medications*—Desmopressin is given in some cases of nocturnal enuresis, and oxybutynin is given for diurnal enuresis to relieve urgency and frequency from bladder irritability.

4. To monitor edema in a child with MCNS:
   A. Keep careful intake and output records.
   B. Weigh the child daily at the same time of day using the same scale.
   C. Measure abdominal girth (every shift).
   D. Watch for signs of respiratory distress, hypertension, or circulatory overload.

5. Hemodialysis removes waste products from the blood by circulating the blood out of the body and into a dialyzer. Waste products are filtered out of the blood through a semipermeable membrane in the machine, and the blood is then returned to the body. The child receiving this type of dialysis must be monitored closely for symptoms related to rapid changes in fluid and electrolyte balance. This pro-

cedure is usually performed three times a week, with each treatment lasting 3–4 hours.

Peritoneal dialysis removes waste products by introducing a chemical solution into the peritoneal cavity and then draining it out again after 4–6 hours. The child may not experience problems of rapid fluid and electrolyte shifts; however, other potential complications include peritonitis, pain, leakage of fluid, and respiratory symptoms. This procedure is usually performed four to six times a day.

6. Suspect peritonitis if the dialysate is cloudy when drained; if the child complains of abdominal pain, tenderness, fever, or constipation; or if the child has evidence of leukocytosis.

7. During the acute phase of APIGN, it is a challenge to increase a child's appetite. Encourage parents to bring favorite foods from home, serve foods in portions that are appropriate to the child's size, maintain a meal schedule similar to that at home, and allow the child to eat with other children or with family members.

8. Corticosteroids are given to reduce inflammation and reverse many symptoms of renal disorders. Side effects, which are common, include moon face, increased appetite, increased hair growth, abdominal distention, and mood swings (cushingoid changes). Children who are taking corticosteroids are at greater risk for infection because these drugs suppress immune function and may mask signs of infection. Extra caution is needed to prevent infection (e.g., avoiding exposure to people who are ill, proper handwashing). To prevent withdrawal symptoms (fever, malaise), the drug dosage is gradually decreased over several weeks. If the child is still receiving immunizations, instruct the parents to wait at least 3 months after the steroids have been discontinued before scheduling an immunization. Otherwise the immunization may not be effective.

Critical Thinking: Application/Analysis

MULTIPLE CHOICE

1. C. For the bladder to empty, the internal and external sphincters must relax while the bladder con-

tracts. Children under 2 years of age have insufficient nerve development to perform these functions.

2. A. The inside of the bladder is exposed through a hole in the outer abdominal wall. Urine continually flows from the ureters onto the abdominal skin, causing skin breakdown.

3. D. The foreskin tissue is used when the urethral defect is repaired.

4. A. Hydronephrosis results when there is an accumulation of urine in the renal pelvis as a result of an obstructed outflow. Relief of the obstruction is necessary for proper function of the kidney.

5. C. The urethra in young girls is very short (2 cm) and is close to the anus, which increases the risk of fecal contamination.

6. D. Cranberry juice appears to inhibit bacterial adherence to the bladder wall and alters urine pH, decreasing the risk of infection.

7. B. Many children who have enuresis have a positive family history, and this is one of the first questions asked in a patient history.

8. B. The protein loss in the urine is a primary indicator of MCNS.

9. A. When protein (albumin) is given intravenously, the oncotic pressure in the blood stream is raised, allowing the fluid in the tissues to flow by osmosis into the vascular compartment. This expands the blood volume and decreases edema in the tissues. This effect is temporary.

10. B. In MCNS the kidneys are working to retain sodium and water, which is adding to the edema. A "no-added-salt" diet will help to control the generalized edema.

11. A. In renal failure the kidney is unable to excrete wastes and concentrate urine. Because potassium is not adequately excreted in the urine,

hyperkalemia occurs. This imbalance can cause serious electrical changes in the heart. Hyponatremia and hypocalcemia also occur because of the impaired excretion and reabsorption of electrolytes.

12. C. Kayexalate removes potassium by exchanging sodium for the potassium in the large intestine. It is given with a laxative, which results in excretion of the potassium in the stool, thereby decreasing the total amount of potassium in the body.

13. C. A complication of hemodialysis is rapid fluid and electrolyte shifts. Hence, monitoring of intake and output is important. Vital signs, blood pressure, and predialysis and postdialysis weight are all measured to monitor fluid balance.

14. D. Children with acute renal failure are susceptible to infection because of altered nutritional status, compromised immunity, and numerous invasive procedures.

15. A. Children with renal failure are at risk for malnutrition because of a high metabolic rate. Depending on the degree of renal failure, sodium, potassium, and phosphorus may be restricted.

16. B. Medication dosages are adjusted to prevent a toxic buildup of the medications in the blood stream. Blood levels of various drugs may be obtained periodically.

17. B. Hematuria occurs as a result of damage to the glomerular membrane. This damage is caused by the deposition of antibody–antigen complexes in the glomeruli, which leads to inflammation and obstruction.

18. B. The testis functions properly at temperatures cooler than 98.6°F (37°C). If it remains in the abdomen, the testis will not produce sperm and will be sterile.

19. A. The child must be monitored for possible infection. The scrotum and groin area will have surgical wounds that must be kept clean. Parents

should be instructed to notify the physician of any redness, warmth, swelling, or discharge from the wound.

20. C. A hydrocele is a fluid-filled mass in the scrotum. In transillumination a light is placed against the skin of the scrotum. If a fluid-filled mass is present, the scrotum will glow from the light in the fluid. If a solid mass is present, the light will be visible only near the source.

21. B. A hydrocele is often associated with an inguinal hernia. If a hydrocele is large, bowel may slip into the inguinal canal and become incarcerated.

CASE STUDIES

1. Yolanda's infection probably began as a urinary tract infection that traveled from the bladder up her ureter to her left kidney. The bacteria that caused the infection is normally found in the bowel, and it is common for young girls to contaminate their urethra with stool.

   To prevent future urinary tract infections, instruct Yolanda to:
   A. Always wipe from front to back after voiding and bowel movements.
   B. Drink plenty of fluids.
   C. Avoid holding urine and waiting to go to the bathroom.
   D. Wear cotton underwear that is not too tight.
   E. Avoid taking bubble baths. They are very irritating to the urethra.
   F. Urinate after intercourse if sexually active.

2. Michael must be interviewed carefully to obtain a complete history with emphasis on his sexual history. He must be reassured that all information he provides will be confidential and that his parents will not be informed. Information that is gathered should include sexual activities, number of partners, use of protective devices (condoms), and the possibility of abuse.

   Treatment of the infection involves completing a full course of antibiotics with follow-up cultures 4–7 days after treatment. Inform Michael that his partners need to be treated as well, because gonorrhea can cause sterility and other complications. They will also receive confidential treatment and counseling. Education about preventing future sexually transmitted diseases includes:

A. Limit the number of sexual contacts.
B. Always use a condom for vaginal and anal intercourse.
C. Refrain from oral sex.
D. Reduce high-risk sexual behaviors.

17

ALTERATIONS IN EYE, EAR, NOSE, AND THROAT FUNCTION

Chapter Overview

Chapter 17 focuses on alterations in eye, ear, nose, and throat function. The anatomy and physiology of pediatric differences for each structure are discussed. Disorders of the eye and ear are presented including infections, visual and hearing disorders, and injuries to the eye and ear. Next, disorders of the nose and throat including epistaxis, tonsillitis, and tonsillectomy are discussed.

Learning Objectives

After studying this chapter, you should be able to:
- Identify normal variations in the eye, ear, nose, and throat in the pediatric population.
- Discuss medical and nursing management of children with infections of the eye.
- Describe selected visual disorders and their treatment.
- Describe the clinical manifestations of children with visual impairments.
- Discuss the emergency care of children with selected eye injuries.
- Summarize the etiology of otitis media and the medical and nursing management of children with this disorder.
- Describe the clinical manifestations of children with hearing impairments.
- Differentiate between conductive and sensorineural hearing loss.
- Discuss the emergency care of children with selected ear injuries.
- Describe the nursing assessment and management of children with epistaxis.
- Describe the medical and nursing management of children with strep throat and tonsillitis.

Review of Concepts

MATCHING

Match the items in list 1 with the appropriate word or phrase in list 2. (*Note:* Items may be used more than once.)

1. Visual Disorders

LIST 1
A. Strabismus
B. Amblyopia
C. Cataracts
D. Glaucoma

List 2

1. ____ Opaque lens
2. ____ Reduced vision in one or both eyes
3. ____ Halos around objects
4. ____ Esotropia
5. ____ Patching of good eye (occlusion therapy)
6. ____ Contact lens postoperatively
7. ____ Distorted red reflex
8. ____ Photophobia

2. Clinical Manifestations of Visual Impairment

List 1

A. Infant
B. Toddler and older child

List 2

1. ____ Bumps into objects
2. ____ Squints
3. ____ Does not imitate facial expressions
4. ____ Holds objects close
5. ____ Is unable to follow an object

3. Causes of Hearing Disorders

List 1

A. Conductive hearing loss
B. Sensorineural hearing loss

List 2

1. ____ Ototoxic drugs
2. ____ Impacted cerumen
3. ____ Foreign body in auditory canal
4. ____ Loud noises
5. ____ Otitis media
6. ____ Maternal rubella

4. Clinical Manifestations of Hearing Impairment

List 1

A. Infant
B. Toddler and preschool child
C. School-age child and adolescent

List 2

1. ____ Speaks in a monotone
2. ____ Babbles little
3. ____ Communicates through gestures
4. ____ Has diminished or absent startle reflex to loud sound
5. ____ Answers questions inappropriately
6. ____ Performs poorly in school or is truant

SHORT ESSAY

1. Outline the anticipatory guidance you would give to a parent about preventing ear infections in infants.

2. A 2-year-old child is diagnosed with infectious conjunctivitis. What instructions would you give to the parents about home care?

3. How would you test an infant's vision?

4. Discuss interventions that would foster normal growth and development in a child with visual impairment.

5. A 10-year-old child who is blind is admitted to the hospital. What factors would you adjust or change in your care of this child?

6. Describe the guidance you would give a parent about cleaning a toddler's ears.

Critical Thinking: Application/Analysis

MULTIPLE CHOICE

Select the best answer.

1. The mother of a newborn tells you that she is very concerned because her baby's eyes do not always move together. The appropriate response is:

A. "This lack of coordination, which is called strabismus, must be corrected with patches."
B. "The eye muscles should become more coordinated by the age of 3 months."
C. "The eye muscles are unbalanced and will require surgery by 2 years of age."
D. "A newborn is unable to focus on objects and will not develop this ability until 6 months of age."

2. A 2-month-old infant can become seriously ill with nasopharyngitis because young infants:

A. Are unable to blow their noses
B. Swallow all sputum and secretions
C. Breathe only through their noses
D. Are unable to cough well

3. Periorbital cellulitis, an infection of the eyelid and tissues surrounding the eye, is:

A. A serious infection requiring vigorous IV antibiotic treatment
B. A viral infection that will resolve on its own
C. Caused by conjunctivitis and treated with antibiotic eye ointment
D. An infection that can result in glaucoma

4. A child has fallen into a bush covered with thorns. One thorn has penetrated the eye. The appropriate first aid at the scene before transporting the child to the hospital is to:

A. Pull thorn from eye to prevent further damage
B. Break off end of thorn to allow eye to close, and cover both eyes
C. Have child carefully hold thorn while you patch eye
D. Leave thorn in eye, cover pierced eye with shield (e.g., paper cup), and cover other eye with patch.

5. Retinopathy of prematurity is associated with:

A. Phototherapy
B. Glaucoma
C. Oxygen therapy
D. Cataracts

6. A bulging tympanic membrane is an indication of:

A. Perforation of tympanic membrane
B. Acute otitis media
C. Thickened tympanic membrane
D. Strep throat

7. Children with otitis media are treated with a full 10- to 14-day course of antibiotics. It is important to instruct the parents to:

A. Give all medication prescribed
B. Give medication until pain is gone
C. Give medication with meals only
D. Ask physician for prophylactic antibiotics

8. Patient education after myringotomy and insertion of tympanotomy tubes would include:

A. Use ear plugs when swimming to keep ears dry
B. Avoid loud noise because ears are more sensitive
C. Flush ear canal gently with water each day
D. Schedule surgery within 6 weeks to remove tubes

9. The hearing of a preschool-age child can be easily assessed by:

A. Having child repeat whispered words
B. Observing whether loud noises startle child
C. Clapping hands near each ear
D. Evaluating language development

10. Teenagers are at risk for permanent hearing loss if they:

A. Develop "swimmer's ear"
B. Have impacted cerumen in canal
C. Drive cars without mufflers
D. Listen to loud music

11. A teenage soccer player collides with another player, hitting the side of his head flat against the other player's chest. He complains of pain in his ear, but there is no drainage in the ear canal. Your advice would be to:

A. Report any dizziness or light-headedness to physician
B. Go home; since there is no drainage, there is no damage to ear
C. See physician only if pain persists next day
D. See physician to rule out ruptured tympanic membrane

12. When speaking to a child with a hearing loss it is important to:

A. Clap hands loudly to get attention
B. Have child's eyes focused on your face and lips
C. Write down all that you say
D. Speak louder than normal

13. To maintain nasal patency in a 2-month-old infant with a cold, you would:

A. Give antihistamine as needed
B. Instill normal saline solution nose drops every 3 to 4 hours
C. Suction nares with bulb syringe every 20 minutes
D. Give decongestant as needed

14. A strep throat is diagnosed by:

A. Throat culture for organism
B. Blood test for organism
C. Presence of lymphadenopathy
D. Appearance of tonsillar exudate

15. Completing the full course of antibiotics for a strep throat infection is very important because an untreated strep infection may lead to:

A. Adhesions in throat
B. Rheumatic fever
C. Tonsillitis
D. Vocal cord damage

16. Which of the following findings would suggest that a child is a candidate for a tonsillectomy?

A. Resistance to antibiotics
B. Chronic otitis media
C. Obstructed breathing

D. Frequent mild sore throats

17. Bleeding after a tonsillectomy is most likely to occur within the first 24 hours and again between:

A. 24 and 48 hours
B. 3 and 4 days
C. 7 and 10 days
D. 2 and 3 weeks

CASE STUDIES

1. 16-year-old Jason spontaneously developed a severe nosebleed. After 10 minutes of trying to stop the bleeding, he informed his parents, who transported him to the emergency department. He has a steady trickle of blood coming from both nares, and the flow goes down his throat when his nares are pinched below the nasal bone. What care would Jason require, and what discharge instructions would be appropriate?

2. Emily, 5 years old, has undergone a tonsillectomy and adenoidectomy. She is receiving intravenous fluids, and her emesis contains dark red blood clots. Emily refuses to drink any liquids or oral pain medication and is drooling saliva. Outline a teaching plan for Emily's parents during the immediate postoperative period and after discharge.

Suggested Learning Activities

1. Formerly, children who underwent tonsillectomy were hospitalized for 1 or 2 days postoperatively and sent home when their condition was stable. Recent changes in insurance reimbursement have resulted in many children being admitted on the day of surgery and discharged the same day.
    A. Visit the utilization review department in your local hospital, and investigate:
        (1) What is their normal stay for a tonsillectomy?
        (2) What complications have occurred?
        (3) What is the readmission rate after tonsillectomies?

B. Interview a surgeon who performs tonsillectomies. Investigate his or her preference regarding length of patient stay, indicators for performing surgery, and minimum age for undergoing the procedure.

2. Public laws require that each state provide educational and related services for handicapped children. Contact a public school in your area and determine how this law is being implemented for children with visual or hearing impairments. What adaptive equipment is available? Are affected children mainstreamed into the classroom? Are resource teachers or tutors available for these children?

ANSWERS WITH RATIONALES

Review of Concepts

MATCHING

1.

1. C	2. B, C, D	3. D
4. A	5. A, B	6. C
7. C	8. D	

2.

1. B	2. B	3. A
4. B	5. A, B	

3.

1. B	2. A	3. A
4. B	5. A	6. B

4.

1. B, C	2. A	3. B
4. A	5. C	6. C

SHORT ESSAY

1. Infants have shorter, wider, and more horizontal eustachian tubes connecting the middle ear to the throat. When an infant sucks or yawns, the eustacian tube valve in the throat is opened. If the infant is fed in a supine position, formula can be swept up into the eustachian tube, causing a middle ear infection. Instruct the parents to hold the infant in their arms with the head up during feeding, and to avoid placing the infant supine in bed with a propped bottle.

2. A. Infectious conjunctivitis is very contagious and can be spread to other family members. Measures to help prevent its spread include careful handwashing after any contact with the child, using washcloths only once before laundering, and preventing other family members from sharing towels with the infected child.

   B. Antibiotic eye ointment or eye drops must be given carefully. (Injury to the eye may occur when giving opthalmic medications if the child is poked by the dispenser tip.) Have the parent demonstrate how to give the medication. Proper cleansing of the eye is necessasry before administering the medication. The eye needs to be washed carefully with water and a cotton ball or washcloth.

   C. The child should be discouraged from rubbing the eye. Applying mittens may be helpful. It is also helpful to keep the child busy and distracted.

3. Infants who are only a few hours old are able to focus on objects and will watch the face intently. Slowly move your face horizontally to see if the infant follows you. Be sure not to make any sound when moving. A brightly colored toy can also be used. Be sure to perform this test several times when the infant is alert and awake. Suspect visual impairment if a 3- to 4-month-old infant does not begin to imitate facial expressions such as smiling, does not make eye contact, or has a dull, vacant stare. Every infant's vision should be assessed.

4. The visually impaired child requires contact with other children as well as sensory input for normal development to occur. To accomplish this, parents need to plan early, regular social activities with other children, encourage self-feeding activities, and provide an environment rich in sensory input to all other senses to compensate and provide adequate sensory stimulation. Some sensory experiences would include stroking, rocking, and hugging, as well as singing and talking to the child.

5. A blind child must be oriented carefully to the room with attention to the placement of objects and the location of the sink, bathroom, and call system. No rearranging of objects should occur unless the child is warned in advance. When entering the room, always announce your presence to avoid startling the

child. The contents of meal trays need to be explained and food positions related to a clock. Be sure that hot objects, such as hot drinks, are identified. When walking with a blind child, walk slightly ahead, and have the child hold your arm to sense your movements. The child needs to be encouraged to be as independent as possible, for example, by going to the playroom alone.

6. Children have cerumen or ear wax buildup just as adults do. Many parents want to clean the child's ear with a cotton-tipped swab. Emphasize the danger of inerting any object, including these swabs, into the ear canal and suggest they not be used. It is possible to rupture the tympanic membrane and injure the middle and inner ears with such a swab. Also, the child may try to mimic the parent by putting a swab into the ear, causing severe damage. Advise the parents to clean the outer ear, only, using a washcloth on the tip of a finger, and washing only those areas that can be reached in this manner.

Critical Thinking: Application/Analysis

MULTIPLE CHOICE

1. B. The extraocular muscles of the eye, including the rectus muscle (responsible for binocular vision), are often not coordinated at birth. A "wandering eye" is often noted by the parent with concern. Although this condition usually resolves completely within 3 months, some infants require future treatment.

2. C. Infants are obligatory nose breathers, and whenever the nasal passages are blocked, normal air exchange is impaired. Mucosal swelling and exudate may block an infant's nasal passage.

3. A. Periorbital cellulitis is a serious bacterial infection that can spread to the optic nerve if not treated promptly with IV antibiotics.

4. D. An object that penetrates an eye should be removed only by a physician. The pierced eye must be protected by covering it with a rigid shield. Both eyes are patched to stop movement of the injured eye, since the eyes move together.

5. C. Retinopathy of prematurity results from injury to the developing capillaries of the retina. Oxygen therapy is associated with its development along with a variety of other factors (e.g., respiratory distress, artificial ventilation, apnea, infection).

6. B. A red, bulging tympanic membrane is a sign of acute otitis media. The lining of the eustachian tube becomes edematous, obstructing the drainage of fluid from the middle ear. The air in the area is absorbed into the blood stream, and fluid from the mucosal lining accumulates, providing an excellent medium for bacterial growth. An ear infection results with a buildup of fluid and purulent material, causing the bulging of the tympanic membrane.

7. A. Children with otitis media need to finish the entire course of medication to eradicate the infection. If the course of treatment is shortened, the infection may recur. Recurrent or chronic otitis media can result in damage to both the inner and middle ear and possible hearing loss.

8. A. During myringotomy, tympanotomy tubes are inserted into the tympanic membrane. These tubes stay in place for several months, and usually fall out spontaneously. They allow air and fluid to flow from the middle to the outer ear and also allow water to flow in the opposite direction. To avoid introducing bacteria directly into the middle ear, the child should wear ear plugs when swimming.

9. A. Preschool children are easily frightened. Whispering is not threatening, can be comfortably performed, and assesses the ability to hear soft sounds.

10. D. Listening to loud music with headphones or at rock concerts is a frequent cause of hearing loss among teenagers and young adults.

11. D. A blow or "slap" injury involving a sudden gush of air against the tympanic membrane can cause the membrane to rupture. The tear can be small or large. If the tear is very small or if there is only air behind the tympanic membrane, there may be no noticeable drainage.

12. B. Many children are taught to read lips and must be looking at your face and lips. Speak at a normal rate and tone and use facial expressions to show caring or concern.

13. B. Saline solution nose drops help to liquefy secretions, which can then be easily removed or swallowed by the infant.

14. A. Diagnosis of strep throat is confirmed by identifying the organism in the throat culture.

15. B. Rheumatic fever can develop after an untreated streptococcal infection. This can result in permanent cardiac damage.

16. C. Tonsillectomy is not routinely performed, but it is indicated when a child has repeated infections with cervical adenitis or chronically hypertrophied tonsils that obstruct breathing and swallowing.

17. C. If the scar that is forming is disrupted, heavy bleeding may occur 7 to 10 days after a tonsillectomy.

CASE STUDIES

1. A. Care during a nosebleed begins with assessment of the blood flow. How much blood is present? Where is it coming from? How long has the patient been bleeding? All tissues and basins of blood are kept to estimate blood loss. Vital signs are assessed frequently to monitor for excessive blood loss.

   Jason should be positioned sitting upright and leaning forward so the blood will not trickle down his throat. He should be instructed to blow his nose forcefully to remove any clots, because the bleeding may be coming from beneath them and pressure over the area may be ineffective until the clots are removed. A pinching pressure should be applied to both nares just below the nasal bone. If blood continues to flow after 10 minutes of pressure, Jason should be instructed to blow his nose again. If the epistaxis continues, the pressure might be reapplied, or a cotton ball soaked in Neo-Synephrine might be inserted to cause vasoconstriction.

   If the bleeding ceases, the area should be examined, and the site cauterized with silver nitrate, if necessary. If bleeding continues, one or both nostrils may need to be packed with petrolatum-impregnated gauze. The packing will remain in place 1 to 7 days. Hematocrit and hemoglobin levels should be checked if significant blood loss has occurred.

   B. Discharge instructions to prevent a future episode of epistaxis would include providing humidification in the teenager's bedroom, discouraging nose picking if this is a problem, moistening the nares with saline solution drops, and applying a thin film of petroleum jelly to the septum twice a day to relieve dryness and irritation. Jason should be instructed to sleep with his head elevated and to avoid bending over, stooping, strenuous exercise, hot drinks, and hot showers or baths for the next 3 to 4 days. Sneezing with the mouth open and blowing the nose gently should also be encouraged.

   Instruct Jason that if a nosebleed should recur, he should assume a forward-leaning position, insert a cotton ball dampened with peroxide or petroleum jelly into the nares, and apply pressure below the nasal bone for 10 to 15 minutes. Ice may also be applied to the bridge of the nose or the back of the neck. After 10 to 15 minutes, the cotton should be gently removed. If the bleeding has not stopped, the physician should be notified.

2. A. Emily has swallowed blood both during and after surgery. Blood is very irritating in the stomach and is often vomited. The dark red color of the blood clots indicates that they are old, so she is not actively bleeding. (Bright red blood clots would indicated recent bleeding, which should

be reported immediately.) Because of the pain in her throat, Emily is refusing to drink. Strongly encourage liquid pain medication, or use nonpharmacologic pain control measures such as an ice collar on the neck or distraction. Oral intake is necessary. All liquids offered should be cool for added comfort. A strategy to improve intake is to offer liquids in 1-ounce measuring cups rather than larger glasses. Crushed ice or popsicles may be more palatable; however, avoid red- or brown-colored items, which might be confused with blood. Avoid using straws, because they create a vacuum in the throat, which could initiate bleeding.

Once the throat pain is controlled, Emily will begin to swallow her saliva. Until then, position her on her side or stomach to allow the drainage to flow from her mouth.

B. Discharge instructions would include the following: (1) continue to give nonaspirin pain medication (aspirin can cause bleeding); (2) encourage Emily to drink cool fluids for several days; (3) avoid rough, scratchy foods for several days; (4) watch for fresh bleeding or vomited blood for the next 7 to 10 days; (5) call the physician if a fever greater than 102°F (38.8°C) develops; (6) chewing gum may help relieve some throat pain, but gum containing aspirin should be avoided; (7) ear pain is expected for several days; (8) although bedrest is not needed, vigorous exercise should be avoided; (9) Emily can return to school after 10 days.

18

ALTERATIONS IN NEUROLOGIC FUNCTION

Chapter Overview

Chapter 18 focuses on alterations in neurologic function in children. Pediatric nervous system differences are presented, and the significance of these differences is explained. Next, altered states of consciousness are described, along with the tools used in neurologic assessments. Seizure disorders, infectious diseases, structural defects, neonatal abstinence syndrome (the drug-addicted infant), cerebral palsy, and injuries of the neurologic system are presented in detail.

Learning Objectives

After studying this chapter, you should be able to:

- Identify significant differences between the adult and pediatric nervous systems.
- Describe the assessment of level of consciousness.
- Describe the use of selected neurologic assessment tools.
- Identify signs of increased intracranial pressure.
- Discuss care of the immobile child.
- Discuss the clinical manifestations of selected seizure disorders and the medical and nursing management of children with these disorders.
- Describe selected infectious diseases that have neurologic implications in children.
- Describe the anatomy and clinical manifestations of selected structural defects of the neurologic system and the medical and nursing management of

children with these defects.
- Discuss identification and care of the infant experiencing neonatal abstinence syndrome.
- Describe the clinical manifestations of cerebral palsy and the medical and nursing management of children with this disorder.
- Describe the etiology, clinical manifestations, and medical and nursing management of head injuries in children.
- Discuss the medical and nursing management of children who have experienced spinal cord injury or near drowning.

Review of Concepts

MATCHING

Match the items in list 1 with the appropriate word or phrase in list 2. (*Note:* Items may be used more than once.)

1. Clinical Manifestations of Seizures

LIST 1
A. Complex partial seizures
B. Simple partial seizures
C. Tonic–clinic seizures
D. Absence seizures
E. Myoclonic seizures
F. Akinetic or atonic seizures

LIST 2

1. _____ Aura may be present
2. _____ Staring
3. _____ Decrease or loss of muscle tone
4. _____ Fluttering of eyelids
5. _____ Paresthesias
6. _____ Grunting
7. _____ Occurs when falling asleep
8. _____ Urinary incontinence
9. _____ Lip smacking
10. _____ Postictal period

2. Characteristics of Cerebral Palsy by Category

LIST 1

A. Hypotonia
B. Hypertonia—Rigidity
C. Hypertonia—Spasticity
D. Athetosis
E. Ataxia

LIST 2

1. _____ Tense, tight muscles
2. _____ Irregularity in muscle coordination or action
3. _____ Floppiness; increased range of motion of joints
4. _____ Scissoring or crossing of the legs
5. _____ Constant involuntary writhing motions
6. _____ Diminished reflex response
7. _____ Exaggerated reflex reactions

3. Head Injuries

LIST 1

A. Concussion
B. Cerebral contusion
C. Intracranial hematoma
D. Cerebral edema
E. Penetrating injury

LIST 2

1. _____ Space-occupying lesion of arterial or venous blood origin
2. _____ Projectile enters the cranial vault
3. _____ Secondary to stretching, compression, or shearing of nerve fibers
4. _____ Increase in intracellular and extracellular fluid in the brain
5. _____ Bruising of brain tissue

SHORT ESSAY

1. Infants have an elastic skull because fontanels and suture lines are open for a period of time after birth. Describe a situation in which this elasticity is an advantage and a situation in which it is a disadvantage.

2. Describe the initial physiologic assessment of a child with an altered level of consciousness.

3. List the signs of increased intracranial pressure that are specific to infants.

4. Children with an altered level of consciousness are at risk of developing complications from immobility such as muscle atrophy, contractures, and skin breakdown. List six nursing measures to prevent these complications.

5. List the manifestations that may occur in the postictal phase of a tonic–clonic seizure.

6. Describe an aura and explain its significance for a child with a seizure disorder.

7. Identify the classes of medications that are frequently given to a child with bacterial meningitis and summarize their effects.

8. Discuss the tests used to diagnose Reye syndrome.

9. Differentiate between communicating and obstructive hydrocephalus.

10. Infants born with a meningocele have surgery within a few days of birth to close the defect. Briefly discuss the preoperative care of these infants.

11. Outline the changes in vital signs that occur in children with head injuries.

12. List the symptoms of a subdural hematoma.

Critical Thinking: Application/Analysis

MULTIPLE CHOICE

Select the best answer.

1. The nerve cells in the nervous system:

    A. Do not increase in numbers after birth
    B. Are completely mature and functional at birth
    C. Are completely replaced by 10 years of age
    D. Continue to increase in number as child grows

2. Which of the following anatomic features makes toddlers more prone to head injuries?

    A. Fontanels and sutures are closed
    B. Abdomen protrudes, with lumbar lordosis
    C. They are unsteady on their feet
    D. Their heads are large in proportion to their bodies

3. A 5-year-old girl who received a head injury in a motor vehicle crash becomes very anxious and agitated while you are assessing her. You would assess her level of consciousness as:

    A. Confusion
    B. Delirium
    C. Stupor
    D. Coma

4. A score of 3 on the Glasgow Coma Scale indicates:

    A. Best level of neurologic functioning
    B. Mild level of neurologic dysfunction
    C. Moderate level of neurologic dysfunction
    D. Total neurologic unresponsiveness

5. An early sign of increased intracranial pressure in an older child is:

    A. Irregular respirations
    B. Fixed and dilated pupils
    C. Headache
    D. Bradycardia

6. The corneal reflex is assessed in an unconscious child by:

    A. Swabbing cornea gently with sterile cotton swab to elicit blink
    B. Shining light source in eye to elicit constriction of pupil
    C. Bringing palm close to eye quickly to elicit blink
    D. Injecting ice water into ear to elicit deviation of eye toward that ear

7. A child with a severely altered level of consciousness may benefit from:

    A. Total quiet environment
    B. Listening to tape of family members talking
    C. Having favorite stuffed animals in bed
    D. Seeing pictures of family and pet

8. A common hallmark of febrile seizures in young children is that they usually occur:

    A. When body temperature falls from high of 39°C (102°F)
    B. With rapid rise in body temperature above 39°C (102°F)
    C. At body temperatures below 38°C (100°F)
    D. When child has no symptoms of illness

9. In a generalized seizure, the airway may be compromised during the:

    A. Clonic phase
    B. Postictal period
    C. Tonic phase
    D. Déjà vu period

10. Staring, inattentiveness, or daydreaming may be signs of:

    A. Simple partial seizures
    B. Absence seizures
    C. Monoclonic seizures
    D. Akinetic seizures

11. A symptom of meningitis in a young infant is:

    A. Change in feeding pattern
    B. Subnormal temperature
    C. Constipation
    D. Generalized floppiness

12. A child in a supine position flexes her knees when her neck is flexed by raising her head. This is:

    A. Positive Kernig sign
    B. Decorticate posturing
    C. Decerebrate posturing
    D. Positive Brudzinski sign

13. To monitor intracranial pressure in a young infant with meningitis, a nurse would evaluate:

    A. Degree of photophobia
    B. Specific gravity
    C. Head circumference
    D. Complete blood cell count

14. A common complication resulting from bacterial meningitis is:

    A. Paralysis
    B. Hearing loss
    C. Vision loss
    D. Cellulitis

15. When a child is diagnosed with meningococcal meningitis, the family and close contacts are:

    A. Hospitalized for treatment
    B. Isolated for 10 days
    C. Treated with prophylactic corticosteroids
    D. Given prophylactic antibiotics

16. Which of the following positions will a child with nuchal rigidity assume for comfort?

    A. Opisthotonic
    B. Fetal
    C. High Fowler
    D. Supine

17. To improve the comfort of a child with meningitis, the nurse should:

    A. Gently rock child
    B. Play musical audio tapes
    C. Keep room lights dim
    D. Massage child's neck and back

18. Follow-up evaluation of children who have recovered from meningitis is important because they:

    A. Need to be treated with prophylactic antibiotics
    B. Need to be monitored for possible complications and sequelae
    C. Have severe psychological problems
    D. Are at high risk for recurrence

19. When viral or aseptic meningitis is suspected, a child is treated with:

    A. Antibiotics
    B. Antiviral agents
    C. Analgesics
    D. No medications

20. Reye syndrome usually develops following:

    A. Bacterial meningitis
    B. Acetaminophen overdose
    C. Strep throat
    D. Mild viral infection

21. Reye syndrome has been associated with the use of:

    A. Ampicillin
    B. Aspirin
    C. Acetaminophen
    D. Pseudoephedrine

22. A nursing priority when caring for a child in the early phase of Guillain-Barré syndrome is:

    A. Keeping child pain free
    B. Continuing active exercise
    C. Monitoring respiratory status
    D. Preventing constipation

23. During the recovery phase of Guillain-Barré syndrome, the priority of care is:

    A. Beginning speech therapy
    B. Recovering lost muscle strength
    C. Fitting child with braces
    D. Preventing excess weight gain

24. Residual neurologic effects in children with encephalitis are:

    A. Rare
    B. Minimal
    C. Common
    D. Preventable

25. The first indication of hydrocephalus in infants is:

    A. Sunsetting eyes
    B. Rapid enlargement of head
    C. Shrill, high-pitched cry
    D. Lethargy

26. An indication of shunt failure in an older child with hydrocephalus is:

    A. Headache upon awakening
    B. Fever and malaise
    C. Head enlargement
    D. Bulging fontanels

27. The child with hydrocephalus has a greater risk of skin breakdown on the:

    A. Sacrum
    B. Scalp
    C. Ribs
    D. Ankles

28. The most serious potential complication following a shunt insertion for hydrocephalus is:

    A. Shunt obstruction
    B. Increased intracranial pressure
    C. Decreased intracranial pressure
    D. Infection

29. After surgical closure of the neural tube defect in a child with myelomeningocele, the priority of care is monitoring for:

    A. Urinary tract infection
    B. Bowel function
    C. Meningitis
    D. Motor function in legs

30. Examination of a child with lower extremity paralysis caused by spina bifida reveals a fractured femur. This fracture was probably caused by:

    A. Blunt trauma
    B. Osteoporosis
    C. Child abuse
    D. Immobility

31. An infant manifesting symptoms of drug withdrawal needs to be monitored closely because:

    A. Symptoms are similar to those of other conditions
    B. Infant is at high risk for sudden death
    C. Hyperglycemia is likely complication
    D. Infant must be properly medicated to achieve optimal comfort

32. One sign of narcotic withdrawal in a neonate is:

    A. Hypotonia
    B. Exaggerated suck
    C. Lethargy
    D. Hyperreflexia

33. Which of the following findings would indicate the need to evaluate an 8-month-old infant for cerebral palsy?

    A. Positive Babinski sign
    B. Asymmetric tonic neck reflex
    C. Uses both hands equally
    D. Not walking

34. A child with cerebral palsy needs a diet:

A. High in calories
B. Low in calories
C. High in iron
D. Low in fiber

35. When a child with cerebral palsy is admitted to the hospital, the plan of care must include:

A. Low-calorie diet because of immobility
B. Bedrest to speed recovery
C. Child's normal exercise program
D. Physical restraints to prevent falls

36. The leading cause of mental retardation, physical disability, and seizures in children is:

A. Head injury
B. Congenital birth defect
C. Cancer
D. Cerebral palsy

37. An infant who exhibits seizures, failure to thrive, vomiting, and lethargy should be evaluated for:

A. Cerebral palsy
B. "Shaken child" syndrome
C. Meningitis
D. Hydrocephalus

38. Which of the following medications are used to shrink brain volume and reduce intracranial pressure?

A. Narcotics
B. Antibiotics
C. Diuretics
D. Corticosteroids

39. The classic signs of a basilar skull fracture are blood behind the tympanic membrane and:

A. Intracranial hematoma
B. Cerebrospinal fluid leaking from nose or ear
C. Pain in posterior skull area
D. Retinal hemorrhage in both eyes

40. To decrease neurologic sequelae, children with spinal cord injuries that result in motor deficits are given:

A. Methylprednisolone
B. Furosemide
C. Ampicillin
D. Diazepam

41. Following spinal cord injury, bladder control may be hard to achieve. The child may need to:

A. Wear incontinence protection
B. Undergo intermittent catheterization
C. Have an indwelling urinary catheter
D. Restrict fluid intake to decrease output

42. The major insult associated with drowning is:

A. Hypoxemia
B. Cardiac arrest
C. Alkalosis
D. Pulmonary edema

CASE STUDIES

1. Eight-month-old Kari fell out of a shopping cart, striking her head. She did not lose consciousness and has cried steadily since the accident. The area above her left ear is swollen and bruised. Kari began to vomit as she arrived in the emergency department. X-ray films show a linear fracture in her left temporal bone. She is admitted for observation for a possible concussion in addition to the fracture. What assessments would be performed on Kari during her hospitalization? Upon her discharge, what instructions should be given to her parents?

2. Amanda, 16 years old, was recently diagnosed with epilepsy after experiencing a tonic–clonic seizure. She is in the 11th grade and is very active in extra-curricular activities. She has begun taking an anticonvulsant and will return to school shortly. Discuss the issues that will cause concern for Amanda and her family and outline an educational plan to meet those issues.

Suggested Learning Activities

1. Many children with severe neurologic disorders are now being cared for at home by family members and home care nurses. Contact a home care nursing agency in your area. Some areas to explore are:

   A. How large is their pediatric caseload? What types of patients are they caring for?
   B. How are the nursing care hours determined?
   C. Is it more difficult to recruit nurses to work with pediatric clients?
   D. How are the services paid for?

2. Contact a head trauma center or rehabilitation center that admits children for rehabilitation after head injuries. Some areas to investigate are:

   A. How are the children evaluated on admission?
   B. What therapies are included in the program?
   C. Are there outpatient as well as inpatient programs?
   D. Are families encouraged to participate in the program?

3. Children who use a wheelchair after a neurologic injury are encouraged to be as independent as possible. The Americans with Disabilities Act, which was signed into law in 1990, contains various deadlines for compliance with its provisions, with a final deadline of 1996 for total compliance. Examine the community in which you live for ease of access to public areas by those with disabilities.

   A. Are public buildings accessible by wheelchair?
   B. Are sidewalks and curbs in good repair and wheelchair-accessible?
   C. Do schools have ramps or elevators to allow full access by students with disabilities?
   D. Are churches and stores accessible?

ANSWERS WITH RATIONALES

Review of Concepts

MATCHING

1.

1. A, C	2. A, D	3. C, D, F
4. D	5. B	6. C
7. E	8. C	9. A
10. C		

2.

1. B	2. E	3. A
4. C	5. D	6. A
7. C		

3.

1. C	2. E	3. A
4. D	5. B	

SHORT ESSAY

1. A. *Advantages:* Open fontanels and sutures allow rapid brain growth during infancy. In conditions in which intracranial pressure is increased, such as hydrocephalus or meningitis, the skull is able to expand, minimizing brain damage.

   B. *Disadvantages:* Open fontanels and sutures place the infant at greater risk for injury from trauma. If such an injury occurs and intracranial bleeding results, the expansion of the skull may mask signs of the bleeding, preventing early diagnosis and treatment. Significant blood loss and pressure on the brain may cause additional injury.

2. The initial physiologic assessment of a child with an altered level of consciousness is:
   A. *Responsiveness*—Assesses response to verbal or tactile stimuli or the environment.
   B. *Airway*—Assesses patency of the airway and methods necessary to maintain it.
   C. *Breathing*—Assesses ventilatory status, color, heart and respiratory rate, respiratory effort, breath sounds, and pulse oximetry or arterial blood gases.
   D. *Circulation*—Assesses heart rate, blood pressure, and capillary refill.
   E. *Disability*—Assesses level of consciousness and response to interventions or environment.
   F. *Exposure*—Assesses body temperature and signs of injury or trauma.

3. The signs of increased intracranial pressure that are specific to infants are bulging fontanels, wide sutures, increased head circumference, dilated scalp veins, and high-pitched, catlike cry.

4. Measures to prevent complications from immobility in children include:
   A. Keeping the body in proper alignment with splints or rolls made from towels or blankets.
      1. Changing the position of the body every 2 hours.
      2. Performing passive range of motion exercises three or four times a day.
      3. Maintaining skin integrity.
   B. Placing the child on a soft bed covering, such as a foam or an egg-crate mattress.
   C. Massaging the child gently with lotion.

5. The postictal phase of a tonic–clinic seizure is characterized by:
   A. Sleepiness and difficulty in arousal
   B. Hypertension
   C. Diaphoresis
   D. Headache, nausea, and vomiting
   E. Poor coordination and decreased muscle tone
   F. Confusion and amnesia
   G. Slurred speech
   H. Visual disturbances
   I. Combativeness

6. An aura is an early sign or warning that may occur when a child is about to have a seizure. The aura may be olfactory or visual in nature; the specific manifestation is unique to each individual. A young child may not recognize the particular sensation associated with an aura; however, careful interviewing may help to identify this warning sign. The child who is able to recognize an aura can take safety precautions, such as lying down to prevent falling, when he or she is about to have a seizure.

7. When treating a child with bacterial meningitis, several classes of medications are given:
   A. *Antibiotics*—Once all diagnostic tests and cultures are performed, antibiotics are begun. Two or three different antibiotics are given to ensure the broadest initial coverage. When the culture results are obtained, the organism causing the infection can be identified, and specific antibiotics can then be prescribed and adjusted so that only the specific drugs that are effective in killing the organism are continued.
   B. *Corticosteroids*—Meningitis may cause the brain to become hyperemeic and swollen. An adrenocorticosteroid is often ordered to decrease the inflammatory response and prevent cerebral edema.
   C. *Anticonvulsants and antipyretics*—Fever is common with meningitis, and acetaminophen (an antipyretic) is the drug of choice to control fever.

8. Reye syndrome is usually diagnosed on the basis of an abrupt change in the child's level of consciousness and on laboratory test results. Liver enzyme levels are elevated to twice normal levels, serum ammonia levels are elevated, blood glucose levels are below normal, and clotting time is prolonged. Liver biopsy, the only study that confirms the diagnosis, reveals fatty deposits in the liver.

9. The types of hydrocephalus are:
   A. *Communicating hydrocephalus*—Involves reduced absorption of cerebrospinal fluid in the subarachnoid space, resulting in a backup of fluid throughout the entire system.
   B. *Obstructive hydrocephalus*—Results from a blockage in the ventricular system within the brain, which prevents the cerebrospinal fluid from entering the subarachnoid space. This type is responsible for 99% of all occurrences in children.

10. Extra care must be taken to prevent the sac from rupturing, which would contaminate the cerebrospinal fluid and place the child at risk for meningitis. Cover the sac with a sterile wet saline dressing to keep the sac from drying out. Place the infant in a prone position with hips slightly flexed and legs abducted to minimize tension on the sac. Maintain this position with towel rolls. Feed the infant with the head turned to one side and give frequent tactile stimulation such as touching, patting, and cuddling. Monitor for motor, bowel, and bladder defects.

11. The vital signs are important indicators of head injury.
    A. *Respiratory*—Changes in effort or periods of apnea can occur because of shock, injury to the spinal cord above C-4, or damage to or pressure on the medulla.
    B. *Heart rate*—Tachycardia can be a sign of blood loss, shock, hypoxia, anxiety, or pain.
    C. *Blood pressure*—Cushing triad, associated with increased intracranial pressure or compromised flow to the brain stem, is characterized by hypertension and increased systolic pressure with wide pulse pressure, along with bradycardia and irregular respirations.

12. Symptoms of a subdural hematoma, which may not appear until 48–72 hours after the injury, include:
    A. Change in level of consciousness (confusion, agitation, or lethargy).
    B. Nausea or vomiting
    C. Headache
    D. Retinal hemorrhages in both eyes
    E. Pupil on side of injury may be fixed and dilated
    F. Seizures
    G. Fever

Critical Thinking: Application/Analysis

MULTIPLE CHOICE

1. A. We are born with all of the nerve cells that we will ever have. If a nerve cell is destroyed, it cannot be replaced.

2. D. Because toddlers' heads are large in proportion to their bodies, they are top-heavy and can easily topple forward. Their neck muscles are not well developed, which adds to their tendency to fall because the neck may not be able to support the large head.

3. B. Delirium is characterized by confusion, fear, agitation, hyperactivity, or anxiety.

4. D. A score of 3 is the lowest possible score on the Glasgow Coma Scale; it indicates total neurologic unresponsiveness.

5. C. In older children, who are able to describe their symptoms, headache is an early sign of increased intracranial pressure. Infants or younger children exhibit nonverbal cues for pain.

6. A. The gentle swabbing of the cornea in an unconscious child should result in a blink if cranial nerves V and VII are intact.

7. B. Because a child who has a severely altered level of consciousness may still be able to hear, talking to the child may be beneficial. An audiotape of family conversations and messages may be soothing to the child and can be played repeatedly.

8. B. Febrile seizures are generalized seizures that often occur when there is a rapid increase in body temperature to temperatures of 39°C (102°F) or above.

9. C. During the tonic phase of a seizure the child loses consciousness, and continuous muscular contractions occur. If the tonic phase is prolonged, the child may be unable to breathe because the respiratory muscles are contracted. This can result in hypoxia.

10. B. Absence seizures (petit mal, lapse seizures) may be difficult to identify because they are usually very brief (5–10 seconds) and do not include the dramatic symptoms (e.g., falling, rigidity, pallor) characteristic of tonic–clonic seizures. Parents or teachers who observe these seizures may not realize that these manifestations are the result of a seizure disorder.

11. A. Many of the symptoms of meningitis in young infants are nonspecific and thus do not alarm parents. A change in feeding pattern such as eating less at each feeding and eating less often is common. The infant may also be feverish, vomit, and have diarrhea.

12. D. A positive Brudzinski sign, which is usually elicited in children with meningitis, indicates the presence of meningeal irritation.

13. C. An infant's fontanels and sutures are not yet fused; therefore, the head circumference will increase if the infant develops an increase in intracranial pressure.

14. B. Most complications from meningitis involve damage to the cranial nerves. The most common complication is hearing loss.

15. D. Meningococcal meningitis is spread by droplet infection and can be easily spread to close contacts. Therefore, all family members and close contacts are treated with a prophylactic antibiotic (rifampin).

16. A. In the opisthotonic position the child lies on one side, the back is arched, and the neck is hyperextended. This relieves some of the discomfort resulting from the meningeal irritation.

17. C. Children with meningitis often have photophobia, and keeping the lights dim reduces this discomfort.

18. B. The child is at risk of developing complications from meningitis. The more common sequelae include hearing loss, attention deficits, seizures, developmental delay, and septic arthritis.

19. A. The child with aseptic meningitis exhibits almost identical symptoms as the child with bacterial meningitis. Therefore, treatment with antibiotics is begun immediately after cultures are taken and continued until aseptic meningitis is confirmed.

20. D. Reye syndrome usually follows a mild viral infection such as varicella, upper respiratory infection, or gastroenteritis.

21. B. The incidence of Reye syndrome has declined since warnings were issued recommending that parents give acetaminophen rather than aspirin to their children. However, the link between aspirin and Reye syndrome is inconclusive.

22. C. Guillain-Barré syndrome results in muscle weakness that begins in the legs and spreads to the trunk, chest, neck, face, and head. The child may experience weakness of the respiratory muscles, resulting in inadequate ventilation that may necessitate intubation and mechanical ventilation. Indicators of inadequate ventilation include fatigue, inadequate effort, color changes, and Pao_2 less than 70 mm Hg.

23. B. Once the progression of weakness and paralysis characterisic of Guillain-Barré syndrome ceases, the child is in the recovery stage. All muscles have lost tone and strength, and an active physical therapy program is begun. This program is continued after discharge.

24. C. Many children are left with neurologic deficits after encephalitis. These deficits include intellectual, motor, visual, or auditory deficits. The cardiovascular system, lungs, and liver can also be affected.

25. B. Because the fontanels and suture lines in the infant skull are open, the increased intracranial pressure of hydrocephalus is first noted in infants by the rapid enlargement of the head.

26. A. The older child's skull is not elastic like that of the infant, so the head is unable to enlarge. Headache resulting from increased intracranial pressure is an indication of shunt failure in these children.

27. B. The skin on the scalp is stretched tightly over the enlarged skull and is at high risk for breakdown, particularly in the area where the shunt catheter is tunneled between the scalp and the skull. Extra care must be taken to cushion the head.

28. D. Shunt infection can occur at any time after surgery but is most prevalent in the first 2 months. Symptoms include ventriculitis, low-grade fever, malaise, headache, and nausea.

29. C. After closure of the defect, it is important to watch closely for symptoms of infection, especially meningitis.

30. D. Children with spina bifida are prone to pathologic fractures of the lower extremities resulting from lack of sensation, immobility, and brittle bones.

31. A. Many of the symptoms seen in drug-addicted infants are identical to those associated with infection, bowel obstruction, hydrocephalus, or intracranial anomaly.

32. D. Drug-addicted infants go through withdrawal after birth. These infants are generally very irritable, jittery, and in constant motion.

33. B. The asymmetric tonic neck reflex should disappear before 6 months of age (see Chapter 3). Its persistence may be an indicator of cerebral palsy.

34. A. The child with cerebral palsy requires a high-calorie diet because of the increased muscle tone. Ensuring sufficient nutritional intake may be difficult, because many children with cerebral palsy have difficult chewing and swallowing. Giving soft foods in small, frequent feedings is often helpful.

35. C. Range of motion exercises are essential to prevent contractures and maintain joint flexibility. The child's usual exercise program must be continued if not contraindicated.

36. A. Head injury is common in children of various ages. Factors that place children at risk for injury include thin cranial bones and unfused sutures, large heads, and impulsiveness. Child abuse accounts for many of these injuries in children less than 1 year of age.

37. B. "Shaken child" syndrome is a form of child abuse in which an infant or child is violently shaken by an adult. The child's brain, moving back and forth inside the skull, can be seriously damaged, sometimes causing death. Adults may shake a child in frustration, assuming this is "better" than hitting the child. However, this behavior can kill or seriously injure a child.

38. C. Diuretics such as mannitol or furosemide may be given to shrink brain volume.

39. B. Cerebrospinal fluid leakage needs to be monitored closely. If leakage persists beyond a week, surgical repair may be necessary.

40. A. Methylprednisolone is administered in high doses. The drug must be started within 8 hours of the injury to achieve maximum anti-inflammatory effect.

41. B. Intermittent catheterization prevents urinary stasis and urinary tract infections.

42. A. Hypoxemia occurs in both wet and dry drowning.

CASE STUDIES

1. Kari is at risk of developing increased intracranial pressure from several possible causes, including intracranial hematoma and cerebral edema. Complete neurologic assessment begins with physiologic assessment (see Table 18–4), Pediatric Glasgow Coma Scale evaluation (see Table 18–3), and cranial nerve assessment (see Table 18–5). These assessments are repeated frequently throughout her hospital stay. If an increase in intracranial pressure is observed, the source of the pressure must be identified and treated. A computed tomographic scan may show a hemorrhage or cerebral edema.

If Kari's condition remains stable, she will be discharged. Discharge instructions for her parents will include signs and symptoms to report to the physician (signs of increased intracranial pressure, changes in level of consciousness, seizures, etc.). Kari's fracture may take up to 6 months to heal completely, and observation should continue throughout that period. Kari's parents should also be counseled about infant safety measures, including use of seat belts in shopping carts and strollers, and use of an approved infant safety seat.

2. A diagnosis of epilepsy is very difficult for both the adolescent and her family to accept. The family will be concerned about the likelihood of subsequent seizures and about how to protect Amanda from injury. Amanda is at a time in her life when the peer group is very important, and she is striving to be accepted by the group. Her concerns will be focused on the possible loss of control over her body movements and loss of consciousness that may occur in front of her friends.

The foremost concern is Amanda's safety. She will not be able to drive, participate in contact sports, or swim unsupervised. She should be instructed to wear a medical alert medallion, either as a bracelet or necklace. The need for Amanda to comply with the medication regimen and avoid skipping any doses must be emphasized. Blood levels of medications will be monitored regularly to ensure Amanda continues to receive a therapeutic dosage. (This is especially important in growing adolescents.) It is also important to emphasize what Amanda can do. Her seizures should be controlled by medication, enabling her to maintain her normal level of activity.

Amanda's parents and teachers need instruction on actions to take if she should have a seizure. The following measures should be emphasized: (1) Do not force anything between Amanda's teeth, (2) turn her on her side, and (3) clear the area of any objects, such as chairs or tables, that might cause injury during the seizure.

Emotional support is very important for both Amanda and her parents. Referral to counseling may be desirable. Community support groups may also be available. Referral to the Epilepsy Foundation of America or Epilepsy Canada can provide the family with more information about epilepsy.

ALTERATIONS IN MUSCULOSKELETAL FUNCTION

Chapter Overview

Chapter 19 focuses on the care of children with alterations in musculoskeletal function. The structural differences between children and adults are discussed. Selected congenital and acquired disorders of the feet, legs, hip, spine, bones, joints, and muscles are presented. Next, musculoskeletal inuries are discussed, with particular emphasis on fractures and their care. Care of children in casts and traction is discussed in detail.

Learning Objectives

After studying this chapter, you should be able to:
- Identify the differences between the adult and pediatric musculoskeletal systems.
- Discuss the clinical manifestations of children with selected disorders of the feet and legs and the medical and nursing care of children with these disorders.
- Describe the clinical manifestations of developmental dysplasia of the hip and the medical and nursing management of children with this disorder.
- Discuss the clinical manifestations of selected acquired disorders of the hip and the medical and nursing management of children with these disorders.
- Identify the classic signs of scoliosis.
- Describe the medical and nursing management of adolescents with scoliosis.
- Discuss the medical and nursing management of children with infections of the bones and joints.

- Describe the genetic transmission and clinical manifestations of osteogenesis imperfecta, and the medical and nursing management of children with this disorder.
- Discuss the genetic transmission and clinical manifestations of selected muscular dystrophies and the medical and nursing management of children with these disorders.
- Discuss the clinical manifestations and nursing management of selected injuries to the musculoskeletal system.
- Describe the care of children in casts and traction.

Review of Concepts

MATCHING

Match the items in list 1 with the appropriate word or phrase in list 2. (*Note:* Items may be used more than once.)

1. Clinical Manifestations of Musculoskeletal Disorders in Children

LIST 1
A. Developmental dysplasia of hip
B. Metatarsus adductus
C. Scoliosis
D. Genu varum
E. Legg-Calvé-Perthes disease
F. Slipped capital femoral epiphysis
G. Talipes equinovarus

List 2

1. _____ Bowlegs
2. _____ Telescoping of thigh
3. _____ Limp; pain in hip or thigh
4. _____ Curvature of lateral border of foot
5. _____ Loss of hip motion
6. _____ Downward and inward direction of foot
7. _____ Lateral curvature of spine

2. Types of Traction

List 1

A. Bryant traction
B. Buck traction
C. Russell traction
D. Dunlop traction
E. Halo traction
F. 90–90 traction
G. External fixators
H. Crutchfield or Vinke tongs

List 2

1. _____ Skeletal traction
2. _____ Skin traction
3. _____ Used for fractured femur
4. _____ Used for cervical fractures
5. _____ Used for fractured humerus
6. _____ Used only for children under 2 years
7. _____ Involves burr holes in skull

SHORT ESSAY

1. Discuss the structural differences between the bones of children and adults.

2. Outline the postoperative assessment and care of a child who has had surgery on the foot and whose leg is in a cast from the knee to the toes.

3. List the common signs and symptoms of developmental dysplasia of the hip (DDH).

4. Explain the process by which slippage of the capital femoral epiphysis occurs.

5. List the neurovascular complications that can occur after spinal fusion for scoliosis.

6. Describe the pathophysiology of osteomyelitis.

Critical Thinking: Application/Analysis

MULTIPLE CHOICE

Select the best answer.

1. Metatarsus adductus ("intoeing") is often treated with:

   A. Surgery
   B. Braces
   C. Stretching exercises
   D. Traction

2. When caring for a child in a wet cast:

   A. Cover cast with absorbent towels
   B. Handle cast only with palms of hands
   C. Dry cast with fan
   D. Avoid touching cast

3. Treatment for clubfoot should begin:

   A. Soon after birth
   B. At 2 months
   C. At 6 months
   D. When child begins to walk

4. The initial treatment of choice in clubfoot is:

   A. Surgery
   B. Stretching exercises
   C. Traction
   D. Serial casting

5. The prognosis for a child with DDH is affected by:

   A. Size of child
   B. Timing of initial treatment
   C. Nutritional status
   D. Presence of other deformities

6. The most common form for DDH in a child under 3 months of age is:

   A. Spica cast
   B. Pavlik harness
   C. Traction
   D. Abduction braces

7. The Pavlik harness should be worn:

   A. At night only
   B. At all times
   C. At least 23 hours per day
   D. During waking hours

8. Legg-Calvé-Perthes disease can result in permanent deformity of:

   A. Midshaft of femur
   B. Hip socket
   C. Distal femur
   D. Femoral head

9. The treatment of Legg-Calvé-Perthes disease is often difficult for school-age children because:

   A. They do not handle pain well
   B. Use of abduction brace limits their activity
   C. They must remain on bed rest for 1 year
   D. School attendance is impossible until treatment is completed

10. The pain that occurs with slipped capital femoral epiphysis can be located in the hip or:

    A. Thigh
    B. Lower back
    C. Lower leg
    D. Iliac crest

11. The population at highest risk for developing scoliosis is:

    A. Girls, 10–13 years of age
    B. Girls, 14–16 years of age
    C. Boys, 10–13 years of age
    D. Boys, 14–16 years of age

12. The hallmark of structural scoliosis is:

    A. Lateral and rotational curvature of spine
    B. Exaggerated curvature of cervical spine
    C. C-shaped curvature of lumbar spine
    D. S-shaped curvature of thoracic spine

13. The normal screening for scoliosis is:

    A. Spinal X-rays
    B. Observation of child's back when bending forward
    C. Observation of child for asymmetric shoulder height
    D. Assessment of leg length

14. A major problem associated with use of a brace in treatment of scoliosis is:

    A. Slowing of child's growth
    B. Constant muscle and bone pain
    C. Patient compliance with wearing brace
    D. Continued progression of curvature

15. Patient education in the treatment of osteomyelitis must emphasize:

    A. Prevention of future infections
    B. Completion of full course of antibiotics
    C. Need for future bone grafts
    D. Care of casted limb

16. Children with osteogenesis imperfecta are often initially suspected of being:

    A. Anemic
    B. Mentally retarded
    C. Clumsy
    D. Battered

17. Which of the following would be contraindicated in a child with osteogenesis imperfecta?

    A. Physical therapy
    B. Walking
    C. Immobility
    D. Swimming

18. A clinical manifestation of Duchenne muscular dystrophy is:

   A. Inability to hold an object
   B. Enlarged calf muscles
   C. Paralysis of lower extremities
   D. Onset after 10 years of age

19. The treatment plan for muscular dystrophy includes:

   A. Exercise
   B. Gait training
   C. Bed rest
   D. High-calorie diet

20. A fracture involving the epiphyseal plate in a child can present added consequences if not treated properly because it:

   A. Places child at greater risk of bone infection
   B. Can increase bone growth in child
   C. Causes higher degree of pain
   D. Can disrupt growth of bone

CASE STUDIES

1. Roberto, who is 9 months old, has DDH. He has just been placed in a spica cast, which extends from his abdomen to both feet. Outline the discharge teaching for Roberto's parents regarding his care.

2. Carolyn, 8 months old, has sustained a spiral fracture of the right femur. Her mother tearfully admits that she twisted Carolyn's leg during a diaper change when the infant would not lie still. Carolyn has been placed in Bryant traction. Adhesive straps are placed on both sides of each leg, and elastic bandages are wrapped around each leg from ankle to thigh. Traction is attached to the adhesive strap at the bottom of the foot. The traction pulls each leg in a perpendicular direction; Carolyn's weight is the counter-traction. Outline a plan of care for Carolyn.

Suggested Learning Activities

1. Visit the pediatric department in your hospital and interview the nurse manager about the types of orthopedic patients cared for in the department. How many children are in traction, casts, or braces? Have they been admitted as the result of injuries or for surgical correction of existing conditions? Review the policies and procedures for caring for pediatric patients in casts and traction.

2. Children may be born without a hand or foot as the result of constrictive amniotic bands in utero. Locate a clinic (e.g., Shriners Hospital) in which these children are treated. Some areas to investigate include:
   A. When is a child first fitted with a prosthesis?
   B. How often are prostheses changed?
   C. How does a prosthetic hand work?
   D. What instructions are given to parents of children with prostheses?
   E. How are these prosthetic devices paid for?

ANSWERS WITH RATIONALES

Review of Concepts

MATCHING

1.
1. D	2. A	3. E, F
4. B	5. F	6. G
7. C		

2.
1. D, E, F, G, H	2. A, B, C, D	3. A, C, F
4. E, H	5. D	6. A
7. H		

SHORT ESSAY

1. The bones of the skull and the long bones of the body demonstrate the significant differences between the bones of children and those of adults. At birth, the cranial bones are connected by a fibrous membrane (fontanels) that allows the skull to grow as well as expand with brain growth. The largest fontanel (anterior) normally closes at 18 months of age. In addition, the ends of the long bones are cartilaginous in children. Replacement of the cartilage cells at the epiphyseal plate by osteoblasts results in the deposition of calcium and bone growth. Injury or disruption of the epiphyseal plate is of great concern in children because further growth of the bone may be impaired. Because the long bones of children are porous and less dense than those of adults, the bones can bend, buckle, or break as a result of a simple fall.

2. Care of a casted leg in the first 24 hours after surgery on the foot would include:
    A. *Neurovascular status checks*—These are performed every 15–30 minutes for the first 2 hours, then every 1–2 hours. The toes are assessed for color, warmth, and edema; capillary refill; sensation to touch; and movement. Distal pulses (if accessible) under the cast are also assessed. Any deviation from normal should be reported.
    B. *Monitoring of postoperative bleeding*—If any bleeding is occurring, it will seep through the batting under the cast to the cast surface. Note the color of the drainage on the cast, draw a line around the area with a ballpoint pen (a felt marker may bleed), and note date and time. If drainage is bright red and copious, notify the physician. If a drainage system (e.g., Hemovac) is in place, monitor the amount of output each shift. If the Hemovac is empty and the drainage on the cast is increasing, the system may be plugged; notify the physician.
    C. *Prevention of edema and pain*—Elevating the casted extremity on a pillow helps to reduce swelling and promotes venous return. Give analgesics routinely in the first 24–48 hours. Note any unexpected increase in pain, and report any pain not relieved by conventional measures.

3. Common manifestations of DDH include limited abduction of the affected hip, asymmetry of the gluteal and thigh fat folds, and telescoping or pistoning of the thigh. Older children walk with a significant limp.

4. A slipped capital femoral epiphysis occurs when the femoral head is displaced from the femoral neck. The slippage occurs along the line of the growth plate, with the bone sliding along that line. Although the cause is unknown, a growth plate abnormality prior to slippage may be a factor. When trauma or chronic weight-bearing stress is added, displacement occurs. The child has a loss of hip motion and mild to severe pain.

5. Possible neurovascular complications from spinal fusion include altered neurovascular status, thrombus formation, paralysis, loss of bowel or bladder control, weakness, and impaired vision or sensation.

6. Osteomyelitis is an infection (bacterial, viral, or fungal) of the bone. The infecting organism can enter the bone by two different routes. It can be spread via the bloodstream, or it can enter the bone directly through a penetrating injury (e.g., stepping on a nail). If the infection is not treated, inflammation and abscess formation may occur, followed by interruption of the blood supply to the underlying bone and, finally, necrosis.

Critical Thinking: Application/Analysis

MULTIPLE CHOICE

1. C. Metatarsus adductus, which is an inward turning of the forefoot, may be related to intrauterine positioning. Simple stretching exercises may correct the problem. If not, serial casting is performed with the foot held in an overcorrected position.

2. B. Care must be taken with a wet cast to prevent indentations (e.g., from fingertips) that could create pressure areas under the cast. A cast can take 24–48 hours to dry.

3. A. Treatment of clubfoot should begin as soon after birth as possible, because the short bones of the foot are primarily cartilaginous at birth but begin to ossify shortly thereafter.

4. D. Casting is begun soon after birth. The foot is manipulated into as correct a position as possible and casted in that position. The casts are replaced every 1–2 weeks because of the infant's rapid growth.

5. B. The longer DDH goes untreated, the more pronounced the clinical manifestations become, and the worse the prognosis.

6. B. The Pavlik harness maintains the infant's legs in a "froglike" position with knees widely abducted. This position reduces the hip dislocation by keeping the femoral head in the acetabulum.

7. C. The Pavlik harness is worn at least 23 hours a day and is removed only for bathing and skin checks.

8. D. The head of the femur becomes necrotic and collapses, losing its normal, rounded shape. If the femoral head is not contained within the hip socket when ossification occurs, the bone will be permanently flattened and misshapen, causing a painful limp.

9. B. The treatment of Legg-Calvé-Perthes disease involves abduction bracing, which forces the legs out to the sides with the knees spread far apart. This bracing severely limits the child's mobility and is particularly difficult for school-age children whose developmental needs include activity and industry.

10. A. The pain in slipped capital femoral epiphysis is often referred to the thigh and/or knee.

11. A. Girls in early pubescence, a period of rapid growth, are at highest risk for developing scoliosis.

12. A. In idiopathic structural scoliosis, the spine curves laterally with vertebral rotation causing a twisting of the trunk. Characteristic findings include uneven shoulders and hips, a one-sided rib hump, and a prominent scapula.

13. B. All school-age children and adolescents should be screened for scoliosis. Children are often screened in school beginning in the 5th grade. For the test the child bends at the waist with arms pointing to the floor. (Refer to Chapter 3.) If the rib cage is higher on one side, the child should be referred for evaluation. The child's siblings should also be examined.

14. C. The brace maintains the existing curvature and prevents any increase but only if worn for 23 hours a day. Compliance with long-term treatment is very difficult for teenagers who are preoccupied with body image.

15. B. Completing the full course of antibiotics is necessary to prevent chronic infection in the bone.

16. D. Children with osteogenesis imperfecta have brittle bones that fracture easily. An X-ray may show old as well as new fractures and may prompt an investigation of child abuse.

17. C. Immobility would further weaken the bones, causing more fractures. Although children with osteogenesis imperfecta need to be handled gently, they must also remain mobile to maintain muscle tone and prevent obesity.

18. B. The calf muscles enlarge because of the infiltration of fat cells in the muscles. Although superficially the child may appear to have strong, well-developed muscles, in reality, they are very weak.

19. A. Muscular dystrophy is a progressive disease. The muscle weakness cannot be reversed; however, efforts are focused on maintaining muscle strength as long as possible, thereby enabling the child to ambulate and preventing joint contractures.

20. D. A fracture in the region of the epiphyseal plate can result in limb length discrepancies, joint incongruities, or angular deformities in growing children.

CASE STUDIES

1. A. *Cast care*—Roberto's cast needs to remain clean, dry, and intact. Because Roberto is still in diapers, you'll need to pay special attention to keeping the perianal area of the cast clean, dry, and odor free. Lining the cast edges with tape provides protection from the raw edges, and the tape can be replaced if it becomes soiled.

   Gently tuck a small disposable diaper into the perianal opening and change it frequently. If the cast should crack, or if any areas begin to get soft, notify the physician. A new cast may need to be applied.

   B. *Skin care*—Avoid using powders and lotions on the skin, particularly in the perianal area. Keep the skin clean and dry. If the cast edges are rough or if pieces of plaster are breaking off, cover the edges with tape. Inspect the skin around the edges often for redness and broken skin. Check inside the top of the cast for stray objects such as toys and food that can cause skin irritation and breakdown.

   C. *Prevention of complications*—It is important to check Roberto's toes several times a day. They should be pink and warm, and he should be able to move them well. If the toes are white or cool, call the physician. The physician should also be contacted if Roberto becomes congested or seems to be having trouble breathing. You'll need to change Roberto's position at least every 2–3 hours when he's awake. He should be placed on his stomach with his toes padded so they are not pressed into the sheets. Laying him on pillows usually works the best. These position changes take pressure off areas under the cast, such as his back and ankles.

   D. *Promotion of normal development*—Provide activities that stimulate Roberto's arms and senses. Be sure to place things within Roberto's reach, but remember that he will place everything into his mouth. Also, avoid small objects that can be hidden inside the top of the cast. Take time to hold and cuddle him and to make him more comfortable.

   E. *Warning signs and symptoms*—Notify Roberto's physician if any of these signs occur:
      1. His toes become cool and white.
      2. He has trouble breathing.
      3. He becomes unusualy irritable and fussy.
      4. He has a sudden, unexpected fever.
      5. New drainage appears on the cast.
      6. The cast becomes cracked, soft, or broken.

   F. *Support*—You'll need to look into sources of help in caring for Roberto. (A referral to a home health care agency should be made.)

2. At 8 months of age Carolyn can sit up, easily turn over, and has begun crawling. Being placed in traction will be difficult for her at this stage of her development. Carolyn's plan of care includes:

A. *Traction care*—The equipment should be checked to ensure that it is in the proper position. The buttocks must be suspended slightly off the bed. The traction weights must hang freely, and the ropes must move freely on the pulleys.

B. *Skin care*—Carolyn's legs must be rewrapped every 4–8 hours, and her skin checked for erythema, edema, and skin breakdown. The adhesive traction straps can cause blisters. They should be removed if a problem is visible. Although her buttocks are off the bed, relieving any pressure on the sacrum, Carolyn's back should be examined periodically, because plastic diaper edges can irritate the skin or small toys scratch or cut the skin.

C. *Neurovascular assessment*—Every 2–4 hours Carolyn's feet should be checked for strength of pedal pulses, warmth, color, capillary refill, movement, and sensation, and any problems should be reported.

D. *Nutrition*—Carolyn is used to sitting in a chair to eat and may have trouble eating solid foods. Her head and shoulders can be raised slightly when she is fed to prevent aspiration.

E. *Mobility*—Carolyn's arms and shoulders will need to be exercised. She should be encouraged to play with age-appropriate toys. Toys can be hung from the overhead traction bar or suspended between the side rails within her reach. Carolyn's natural tendency is to turn over on her stomach, and a jacket restraint may be needed to discourage her. (*Caution:* Any chest restraint can compromise Carolyn's breathing. She must be checked every 30 minutes if restrained. The need to prevent the buttocks from resting on the bed must be considered when deciding if restraint is needed. If there is enough distraction above Carolyn, she will have less interest in turning over.)

F. *Comfort*—After a fracture children often have muscle spasms, which are very painful. Evaluate Carolyn carefully, and administer ordered analgesics and muscle relaxants. Remember that distraction is a nonpharmacologic measure that works well with infants (see Chapter 7).

G. *Psychological development*—Encourage Carolyn's mother to visit and stay with her daughter. Her mother is emotionally stressed and may fear repercussions from the staff because she inflicted the injury. This does not mean, however, that she does not love her daughter. By approaching the mother in a caring, nonjudgmental way, the staff can help her to recognize the stresses that led to the abuse and help her to deal with them positively. Carolyn is very dependent upon her mother at this age, and her mother's presence is needed for her psychological health. (Refer to Chapter 22 for further discussion of nursing care of the abused child.)

20

ALTERATIONS IN ENDOCRINE FUNCTION

Chapter Overview

Chapter 20 focuses on alterations in endocrine function in children. The anatomy and physiology of the endocrine system are reviewed, with a discussion of the role the endocrine glands have in normal development. Disorders of altered pituitary, thyroid, adrenal, and pancreatic function are presented. Medical and nursing management of the child with diabetes mellitus is discussed in detail. Additional topics include disorders of altered gonadal function, disorders related to sex chromosome abnormalities, and inborn errors of metabolism.

Learning Objectives

After studying this chapter, you should be able to:
- Discuss the role of various organs and glands of the endocrine system in the growth and development of children.
- Describe the etiology and clinical manifestations of selected disorders of the endocrine system.
- Discuss the medical and nursing management of children with selected endocrine disorders.
- Outline the medical and nursing management of children with insulin-dependent diabetes mellitus (IDDM).
- Describe the clinical manifestations of sex chromo-

some abnormalities and the medical and nursing management of children with these disorders.
- Identify disorders for which newborn screening is mandated.
- Describe the clinical manifestations of inborn errors of metabolism and the medical and nursing management of children with these disorders.

Review of Concepts

COMPLETION

Describe the cause of the hormone imbalances in the following endocrine disorders.

Disorder	Cause of Imbalance
A. Hypopituitarism	
B. Hyperpituitarism	
C. Diabetes insipidus	
D. Diabetes mellitus	
E. Precocious puberty	

Disorder	Cause of Imbalance
F. Hypothyroidism	
G. Hyperthyroidism	
H. Cushing's syndrome	
I. Congenital adrenal hyperplasia	
J. Addison's disease	
K. Pheochromocytoma	

MATCHING

Match the items in list 1 with the appropriate word or definition in list 2. (*Note:* Items may be used more than once.)

1. Clinical Manifestations of Disorders of Altered Pituitary Function

LIST 1
A. Hypopituitarism
B. Hyperpituitarism
C. Diabetes insipidus
D. Precocious puberty

LIST 2
1. ____ Hypernatremia
2. ____ Short stature
3. ____ Premature sexual development
4. ____ Excessive height
5. ____ Premature skeletal maturation
6. ____ Polyuria and polydipsia

2. Abnormal Serum Glucose Levels

LIST 1
A. Hypoglycemia
B. Hyperglycemia

LIST 2
1. Tachycardia
2. Headache, dizziness
3. Fruity or acetone breath
4. Pallor, sweating
5. Flushed skin
6. Dry mucous membranes, thirst
7. Irritable, nervous
8. Gradual onset
9. Abdominal pain
10. Tremors, shaky feeling

SHORT ESSAY

1. Describe the signs and symptoms of Cushing's syndrome.

2. Discuss the etiology of IDDM.

3. Describe how untreated IDDM causes metabolic acidosis.

4. Using the accompanying diagram of insulin levels over a 24-hour period, answer the following questions:
   A. Why are short-acting (regular) and intermediate-acting (NPH) insulin given together in the morning and evening?
   B. At what times of day would a child be likely to have a hypoglycemic response? What measures are needed to prevent hypoglycemia at these times?
   C. When would a teenage football player be at risk for hypoglycemia?
   D. When would a grade school–aged child be at risk for hypoglycemia?
   E. How would a hypoglycemic reaction at 3 AM be avoided?

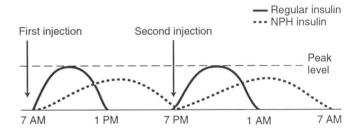

Critical Thinking: Application/Analysis

MULTIPLE CHOICE

Select the best answer.

1. Which of the following findings would lead the clinician to suspect hypopituitarism in a child?

   A. Hyperglycemia
   B. Failure to gain weight
   C. Height 3 standard deviations below mean
   D. Shorter than siblings at same age

2. Early recognition of hypopituitarism is important because:

   A. Early treatment ensures attainment of maximum height potential
   B. Treatment can be given at puberty for growth spurts
   C. Parents are able to plan for expensive treatments
   D. Testing for other disorders is initiated

3. The secretion of antidiuretic hormone (ADH) results in:

   A. Dilution of urine
   B. Concentration of urine
   C. Dehydration
   D. Hypernatremia

4. Children are usually diagnosed with diabetes insipidus when they develop:

   A. Severe hyponatremia
   B. Generalized edema
   C. Congestive heart failure
   D. Severe dehydration

5. Precocious puberty ultimately results in:

   A. Delayed closure of epiphyseal plates
   B. Shortened pubertal development
   C. Excessive height
   D. Premature closure of epiphyseal plates

6. Mandatory newborn screening is performed to identify:

   A. Hypopituitarism
   B. Hyperpituitarism
   C. Hypothyroidism
   D. Hyperthyroidism

7. Untreated hypothyroidism can result in:

   A. Mental retardation
   B. Accelerated growth
   C. Increased appetite
   D. Hypertonia

8. A side effect of the synthetic thyroid hormone levothyroxine (Synthroid) that should be reported is:

   A. Dyspnea
   B. Tachycardia
   C. Hypotension
   D. Generalized edema

9. A classic manifestation found in hyperthyroidism is:

   A. Hypotension
   B. Decreased appetite
   C. Lethargy
   D. Bulging eyes

10. Treatment of hyperthyroidism with radioactive iodine (^{131}I) will result in:

    A. Permanent hypothyroidism
    B. Euthyroid state
    C. Partial inhibition of thyroid hormone secretion
    D. Temporary relief of symptoms

11. After a thyroidectomy the child must be observed postoperatively for:

    A. Immediate hypothyroidism
    B. Hypocalcemia
    C. Thyroid storm
    D. Hypernatremia

12. A newborn girl with congenital adrenal hyperplasia may be born with:

    A. Pseudohermaphroditism
    B. Cushing's syndrome
    C. Addison's disease
    D. Graves' disease

13. Children with adrenal hyperplasia are treated with:

    A. Androgens
    B. Adrenocorticotropic hormone (ACTH)
    C. Hydrocortisone
    D. Estrogen

14. What type of insulin may be used by adolescents to achieve tight glucose control?

    A. Humalog
    B. Regular
    C. NPH
    D. Ultralente

15. A laboratory test that demonstrates compliance with diabetic regimen for the previous 3–5 weeks is:

    A. Glycosylated hemoglobin (HbA$_1$c)
    B. Fasting blood glucose
    C. Two-hour postprandial blood glucose
    D. Glucose tolerance test

16. A child with IDDM is usually given two different types of insulin to:

    A. Increase cell sensitivity to insulin
    B. Avoid daily blood glucose testing
    C. Prevent body from developing resistance to one type
    D. Maintain blood glucose level as close to normal as possible

17. Which age group has the most difficulty dealing with a diagnosis of IDDM?

    A. Toddler
    B. Preschool age
    C. School age
    D. Adolescent

18. Symptoms that may indicate hypoglycemia in a diabetic toddler are:

    A. Irritability and fussiness
    B. Lethargy and sleepiness
    C. Nausea and vomiting
    D. Dry mouth and thirst

19. A boy with gynecomastia needs to be informed that:

    A. Condition is usually temporary
    B. All boys have this breast development
    C. There is no treatment for condition
    D. Surgical treatment is necessary

20. Which of the following factors is a cause of secondary amenorrhea?

    A. Recent change in diet
    B. Sexually transmitted diseases
    C. Excessive physical activity
    D. Turner's syndrome

21. Which of the following medications is most effective in relieving discomfort of dysmenorrhea?

    A. Codeine
    B. Diazepam
    C. Ibuprofen
    D. Dexamethasone

22. Turner's syndrome may not be diagnosed until a child:

    A. Is 6–12 months old
    B. Reaches 5 years of age
    C. Begins to fail in school
    D. Is a teenager

23. Treatment of Turner's syndrome consists of

    A. Growth hormone replacement
    B. Estrogen therapy at puberty
    C. Parathyroid hormone replacement
    D. Androgen replacement

24. Boys with Klinefelter's syndrome are usually:

    A. Highly intelligent
    B. Short in stature
    C. Infertile
    D. Severely mentally retarded

25. A child with galactosemia must avoid eating:

    A. Milk and cheese
    B. Meat and fish
    C. Legumes and oats
    D. Certain vegetables

CASE STUDIES

1. Juanita, 14 years old, was brought to the emergency department by her parents, who were worried by her symptoms of lethargy and confusion. They stated that Juanita had been experiencing gastroenteritis, vomiting, and diarrhea for the past 3 days. Juanita's serum glucose level on admission was 535 mg/dL, and her urine contained large amounts of ketones and glucose. Her arterial blood gas results revealed metabolic acidosis. Juanita's parents stated that their daughter had been complaining of thirst and increased urination for the past 2 weeks, and they noted that she was eating more than usual but had assumed she was in a growth spurt. Juanita is diagnosed with IDDM, and treated for diabetic ketoacidosis (DKA). Outline a discharge plan for Juanita and her parents.

2. Meghan is 1 week old when her parents are notified that the result of her phenylketonuria (PKU) test is positive. After a repeat test confirms the diagnosis, the family is referred for treatment of Meghan's PKU. Describe the cause of PKU and outline the education that will be given to Meghan's family about the disorder.

Suggested Learning Activities

1. Visit the pediatric unit at your hospital or clinic and review a copy of the materials given to children who are newly diagnosed with IDDM. Some areas to review are:
    A. Is there an organized educational plan for these children? How is progress documented?
    B. Is information provided about the following topics: definition and cause of diabetes, insulin administration, blood glucose and urine testing, and diet instruction?
    C. Are families referred to support groups, the American (or Canadian) Diabetes Association, or a home care agency?
    D. How long do children newly diagnosed with IDDM remain in the hospital?

2. Research the types of newborn screening that are mandated in your state.
    A. What disorders are screened for, and how is the screening accomplished?
    B. How are parents notified of the results?

ANSWERS WITH RATIONALES

Review of Concepts

COMPLETION

Hormone Imbalances in Endocrine Disorders

Disorder	Cause of Imbalance
A. Hypopituitarism	Deficiency of growth hormone
B. Hyperpituitarism	Excess of growth hormone
C. Diabetes insipidus	Deficiency of antidiuretic hormone
D. Diabetes mellitus	Disorder of glucose metabolism
E. Precocious puberty	Early stimulation of pubertal hormones
F. Hypothyroidism	Deficiency of thyroid hormones
G. Hyperthyroidism	Excess of thyroid hormones
H. Cushing's syndrome	Excess of glucocorticoids
I. Congenital adrenal hyperplasia	Deficiency of enzymes needed for cortisol production
J. Addison's disease	Deficiency of glucocorticoids and mineralocorticoids
K. Pheochromocytoma	Tumor of the adrenal medulla

MATCHING

1.
1. C	2. A, D	3. D
4. B	5. D	6. C

2.
1. A	2. A	3. B
4. A	5. B	6. B
7. A	8. B	9. B
10. A		

SHORT ESSAY

1. Cushing's syndrome results from excess levels of glucocorticoids (secreted by the adrenal glands) in the bloodstream. The initial sign in most children is gradual generalized obesity and growth retardation. It takes up to 5 years for the child to develop the characteristic "cushingoid" appearance—moon face (chubby cheeks and a double chin) and fat pads over the shoulders and back (buffalo hump). Other signs and symptoms include hypertension; weight gain with distribution primarily on the trunk; striae on the abdomen, buttocks, and thighs; fatigue; muscle weakness and wasting; acne; bruising; osteoporosis; growth failure with delayed bone age; and mental changes and delayed puberty.

2. Three factors play a role in the onset of IDDM:
   A. *Genetic*—There is a strong familial tendency with no specific pattern of inheritance. The child inherits a susceptibility to the disease rather than the disease itself.
   B. *Environmental*—Viruses or chemicals in the diet are believed to play an important role in damaging the beta cells in the islets of Langerhans (insulin-producing cells).

C. *Autoimmune response*—The body has an immunologic response to an inflammatory process as evidenced by circulating antibodies in pancreatic islet cells. As the beta cells are destroyed, the level of circulating antibodies falls.

3. In IDDM the majority of the beta cells in the pancreas are destroyed. This dramatically decreases the production of insulin, which helps to transport glucose into the cells. Lack of insulin, therefore, results in a rise in blood glucose levels and a decrease of glucose in the cells. Glucose is a necessary source of energy for the cells. The body, unable to use glucose for metabolism, turns to an alternate source of energy—free fatty acids. When these acids are metabolized by the liver, however, ketone bodies are produced as a by-product. Accumulation of ketone bodies in the body results in metabolic acidosis or ketoacidosis.

4. A. Regular (short-acting) and NPH (intermediate-acting) insulin are given together because the differences in their onset of action and peak activity ensure that a fairly consistent level of insulin is present in the bloodstream for at least a 12-hour period. Regular insulin begins to act within ½–1 hour of injection, NPH between 1 and 2 hours after injection. When both forms are given before a meal, the regular insulin is active when the meal is consumed, peaking after 2–4 hours. The NPH acts more slowly. Thus, as the regular insulin activity is dropping, the NPH activity is reaching its peak. With this regimen the child requires only two injections per day instead of four or more to regulate the absorption of glucose.

B. Hypoglycemia occurs when there is insulin in the bloodstream but not enough glucose available for it to act on. A child is most vulnerable to hypoglycemia when the insulin is at peak activity and not enough food has been consumed. Midafternoon is one such time. Assume that a child has lunch around 11AM or 12 noon. Because the NPH insulin activity peaks around 3 PM, the child will need to eat a snack at midafternoon to cover the peak of the NPH insulin. (If the child has eaten a snack and still has a hypoglycemic response, the physician

should be notified. A decrease in insulin dosage may be necessary.)

C. Because regular exercise increases insulin sensitivity and improves metabolic control, less insulin may be needed. Athletes are at risk during afternoon practice and game times because the NPH insulin activity is peaking at that time. They need to test their blood glucose levels before, during, and after their first few practices and to eat snacks as needed to maintain an appropriate blood glucose level.

D. A grade school–aged child would be at risk for a hypoglycemic reaction midmorning while at school and midafternoon while traveling home from school. For this reason school bus drivers should be informed of any children with IDDM who ride the bus.

E. The 3 AM peak of NPH insulin activity needs to be covered with an evening snack that is high in protein. If this snack does not cover the 3 AM peak, the dosage of NPH insulin may need to be reduced. A severe reaction at this time can be very dangerous because the child and family are asleep and are unaware of the reaction. Without appropriate treatment brain damage can occur.

Critical Thinking: Application/Analysis

MULTIPLE CHOICE

1. C. The pituitary gland secretes growth hormone. If a child is 3 standard deviations below the mean height for age, investigation into the cause is necessary. Other causes may be familial stature, constitutional growth delay, skeletal dysplasias, or psychosocial dwarfism.

2. A. Early treatment with growth hormone helps the child attain maximum height potential. Treatment should start in early childhood because the synthetic hormone stimulates the growth of all body tissues.

3. B. Antidiuretic hormone facilitates concentration of the urine by stimulating reabsorption of water from the distal tubule of the kidney.

4. D. The child with diabetes insipidus is constantly thirsty. The child attempts to satisfy thirst by drinking large quantities of water; however, body fluids are depleted because, without antidiuretic hormone, the kidneys are not stimulated to conserve water. A large volume of dilute urine is excreted, resulting in dehydration.

5. D. Precocious puberty occurs when the normal hormones responsible for pubertal changes are secreted early. The child experiences an early growth spurt and secondary sex characteristics appear. Because skeletal maturation is premature, these children appear very tall for their age. Their growth ceases prematurely, however, because the pubertal hormones stimulate closure of the epiphyseal plates, resulting in short stature at maturity.

6. C. All 50 states mandate screening for hypothyroidism, which has dramatically decreased the number of untreated cases.

7. A. The thyroid hormones are important for growth and development and for the metabolism of nutrients and energy. In untreated hypothyroidism, growth is delayed and mental retardation develops.

8. B. Parents need to be taught how to take their child's pulse and to recognize when it is increased. Tachycardia could indicate the presence of excess thyroid hormone.

9. D. Common characteristics of a child with hyperthyroidism are tachycardia, goiter, bulging eyes, irritability, increased appetite, weight loss, emotional lability, heat intolerance, and muscle weakness.

10. A. Radioactive iodine (^{131}I) destroys the thyroid gland, resulting in permanent hypothyroidism and the need for lifelong hormone replacement.

11. C. Thyroid storm (severe thyrotoxicosis) may occur when thyroid hormone is suddenly released into the bloodstream during surgery. Symptoms are fever, diaphoresis, tachycardia, prolonged shock, and, if untreated, death.

12. A. The fetus with congenital adrenal hyperplasia lacks sufficient production of cortisol by the adrenal gland. As a result, the pituitary gland increases secretion of ACTH. The high ACTH levels cause the adrenal glands to continue to secrete androgens, which results in sexual ambiguity of infant girls at birth. The female genitalia are virilized with an enlarged clitoris and labial fusions. A karyotype (chromosome study) may be obtained to determine the sex of the infant.

13. C. Administration of glucocorticoids (hydrocortisone) results in reduced ACTH secretion and suppression of the excessive androgen production. The child's growth and sexual development are closely monitored.

14. A. Humalog is a rapid-acting insulin that has an onset of 5–15 minutes and peaks in 1 hour. This is helpful for the adolescent who has erratic eating habits particularly with peers (e.g., eating pizza with friends after a movie). A dose of Humalog can be given before the late night meal.

15. A. The hemoglobin molecule normally incorporates glucose into its structure. If the blood glucose level is high, more glucose is attached to the hemoglobin; if it is low, less is incorporated. The glycosylated hemoglobin reflects the average blood glucose over a period of several weeks. This is especially useful when monitoring children who are difficult to regulate or those who have a history of failing to take their insulin or of not following their diet.

16. D. Giving a short-acting insulin and an intermediate- or long-acting insulin before breakfast and before dinner ensures that insulin will be present in the bloodstreasm throughout the day. This helps the body to maintain the serum glucose level as close as possible to a normal level.

17. D. Adolescents often deny having diabetes so they can be like their peers when eating and exercising. Because their complaince with the treatment regimen is often poor, they can experience severe complications such as diabetic ketoacidosis (DKA).

18. A. Parents need to be able to recognize behaviors such as irritability and fussiness that indicate possible hypoglycemia. A blood glucose test should be performed immediately; if the glucose level is low, the toddler should be given a carbohdrate-containing snack or drink.

19. A. Gynecomastia usually disappears in 1–2 years. (In rare cases a simple mastectomy is necessary to remove the excess tissue.)

20. C. Excessive physical activity or sports training can result in the cessation of menses.

21. C. Dysmenorrhea is usually caused by increased secretion of prostaglandins. NSAIDs (e.g., ibuprofen) decrease prostaglandin synthesis and are effective if taken before cramping starts.

22. D. When there are few physical characteristics, diagnosis is made only when short stature and delayed puberty become apparent in the teenage years.

23. B. Girls with Turner's syndrome fail to develop secondary sexual characteristics and have amenorrhea. They are started on low-dose estrogen therapy to stimulate pubertal changes. After 2–3 years progesterone is added to initiate menstrual periods.

24. C. Boys with Klinefelter's syndrome have delayed growth of the testes and require testosterone replacement to stimulate masculinization.

25. A. Infants and children are placed on a galactose-free diet, which excludes milk and cheese products.

CASE STUDIES

1. Adolescence is a difficult period in which to be diagnosed with IDDM. Juanita is striving for independence from her parents, and the peer group is very important in her life. The diagnosis of a chronic illness makes Juanita see herself as different from her peers and raises fears of rejection. This diagnosis is also difficult for Juanita's parents who, in seeking to protect her, may prevent her from becoming independent.

It is important that Juanita be the focus of all teaching. In this way staff members demonstrate their recognition of her need for independence and also make her responsible for her own care. Juanita's parents need to receive the information as well; however, it must be clear that Juanita is the primary learner. Juanita is old enough to understand all aspects of her disease and should be able to perform blood glucose testing and administer her own insulin.

The educational plan in the hospital will initially cover blood glucose monitoring, insulin measurement and administration, urine testing for ketones, and diet instruction. Also covered will be symptoms of hyperglycemia and hypoglycemia and their individual treatment plans. Teenagers are very adept at learning the technical aspects of their treatment plan; however, they often have difficulty complying with the dietary regimen. Teenagers wish to conform to their peer group, and eating is a major social activity among adolescents. With planning and "planned cheating," Juanita can anticipate meals with peers and adapt her diet for the day to accommodate this meal. It is also important to emphasize the importance of sufficient caloric intake each day and the need to avoid reducing diets.

Other areas to discuss include a regular exercise program, which improves insulin sensitivity, and skin care. Juanita needs to wear medical alert identification. The school nurse, teachers, and coaches also should be notified of Juanita's diagnosis and should be informed of what action to take if she has a hypoglycemic reaction.

A referral to a home care nursing agency should be made so that follow-up instruction can be provided, as needed. Juanita and her family have had to absorb large amounts of information in a short time, while they were still in shock from the diagnosis. The home care nurse can reiterate information, assist the family to cope with the diagnosis, help the family to adjust Juanita's regimen into the family routine, and promote Juanita's self-esteem with praise and positive feedback.

2. All infants in the United Sates are screened for PKU 24 hours after birth. PKU is an inherited disorder of amaino acid metabolism that affects the body's utilization of protein. The child with PKU is missing the liver enzyme phenylalanine hydroxylase, which breaks down the amino acid phenylalanine. This deficiency results in an accumulation of phenylalanine in the blood that, if not decreased over a 2- to 3-year period, results in a seizure disorder and mental retardation.

Meghan will require a special formula and a diet low in phenylalanine. Because it is impossible to completely eliminate phenylalaline from the diet, the goal is to keep the blood level between 2 and 8 mg/dL. High-protein foods (meats and dairy products) and aspartame (an artificial sweetener sold under the trade names of Equal and Nutrasweet) are avoided because they contain large amounts of phenylalanine.

Meghan's family needs to understand her dietary restrictions, particularly when she begins eating solid foods. All labels need to be checked for dairy products and aspartame. The diet neds to be maintained until late school age or adolescence, when brain growth ceases. Because this disorder is inherited, Meghan should be referred to a genetic counselor when she reaches child-bearing age and beings planning her family. If she does decide to have a child, she will need to resume a low-phenylalanine diet before conception to prevent congenital defects in the fetus. Meghan's parents should also be referred for genetic counseling if they are considering a future pregnancy.

21

ALTERATIONS IN SKIN INTEGRITY

Chapter Overview

Chapter 21 focuses on the care of children with alterations in skin integrity. The differences between the skin and accessory structures in adults and children are presented. Common pediatric skin problems are discussed, including skin lesions, dermatitis, acne, and infectious disorders. Injuries to the skin are discussed, including pressure ulcers, sunburn, hypothermia, frostbite, bites (animal, human, and insect), contusions, and foreign bodies. Burns are discussed in detail, including types, classification, medical treatment, and nursing management.

Learning Objectives

After studying this chapter, you should be able to:
- Identify the differences between the skin of children and adults.
- Describe common secondary skin lesions.
- Discuss the care of children with dermatitis.
- Describe the cutaneous responses that occur in adverse reactions to drugs.
- Outline an educational plan for a child with eczema.
- Describe the medical and nursing management of children with selected infectious skin disorders.

- Discuss the care of children with cellulitis.
- Differentiate between folliculitis and acne and summarize the care of children with these disorders.
- Describe the medical and nursing management of selected injuries to the skin.
- List the types of burns and the classification of burn severity.
- Calculate the percentage of burn injury using a body surface area chart.
- Discuss the medical and nursing management of a child with major burns.

Review of Concepts

COMPLETION

1. Give an example for each type of secondary skin lesion listed:

Lesion Name	Example
A. Crust	
B. Scale	
C. Lichenification	
D. Scar	

Lesion Name	Example
E. Keloid	
F. Excoriation	
G. Fissure	
H. Erosion	
I. Ulcer	

2. Indicate the site of the infection and the clinical manifestations of the following types of tinea infection (ringworm):

Type	Site	Clinical Manifestions
A. Tinea capitis		
B. Tinea corporis		
C. Tinea cruris		
D. Tinea pedis		

MATCHING

Match the items in list 1 with the appropriate word or phrase in list 2. (*Note:* Items may be used more than once.)

1. Common Burn Injuries by Age Group

LIST 1
A. Thermal
B. Chemical
C. Electrical
D. Radiation

LIST 2
1. ____ Infant
2. ____ Toddler
3. ____ Preschool age
4. ____ School age
5. ____ Adolescent

SHORT ESSAY

1. Compare allergic contact dermatitis with irritant contact dermatitis.

2. What advice would you give to parents of a child with diaper dermatitis?

3. Outline instructions to be given to the parents of a 6-year-old child with head lice.

4. List the three criteria considered when determining burn severity.

5. Compare partial-thickness and full-thickness burns.

6. List the reasons for placing a child with burns in a whirlpool bath.

7. Describe the four types of grafts that are used for burns.

8. Describe the advantages of play therapy for children with burns.

9. List five strategies to protect children from sunburn.

Critical Thinking: Application/Analysis

MULTIPLE CHOICE

Select the best answer.

1. Which characteristic of newborn skin is responsible for the infant having difficulty with heat loss and body temperature regulation? The newborn's skin has:

A. More water than adult's skin
B. Immature apocrine glands
C. Little subcutaneous fat
D. Lanugo on back and shoulders

2. Careful interviewing of parents of an infant with seborrheic dermatitis (cradle cap) often reveals that the parents:

A. Are afraid to wash infant's hair
B. Use harsh adult shampoos on infant
C. Wash infant's hair every day
D. Never oil infant's hair

3. Seborrheic dermatitis that does not occur on the scalp is treated with:

A. Alcohol
B. Mild soap
C. Topical corticosteroids
D. Silvadeen cream

4. Whenever a child is given a prescription for a new medication, the parents should be instructed to:

A. Give medication until child's symptoms disappear
B. Report any rashes, hives, or itching
C. Watch for any change in weight
D. Stop giving drug as soon as child feels better, to avoid dependency

5. Children with eczema often have a history of:

A. Recent viral illness
B. Intolerance of heat or cold
C. Allergies to medications
D. Family history of asthma

6. Measures to decrease skin irritation in eczema would include:

A. Use of mild soap (Dove or Tone)
B. Use of fabric softeners for all clothes
C. Wearing clothing made from natural fibers (e.g., wool)
D. Taking hot baths or showers daily

7. Appropriate advice about skin care for a teenager with acne is:

A. Use astringents to close pores
B. Use deodorant soap to kill germs
C. Avoid touching lesions
D. Break pustules so they will drain

8. Teenagers who are taking vitamin A preparations should be advised to:

A. Avoid exposing skin to sun
B. Avoid eating chocolate
C. Eat low-fat diet
D. Avoid consuming milk products

9. Many adolescents with cystic acne are treated with:

A. Hydrogen peroxide
B. Corticosteroids
C. Astringents
D. Oral antibiotics

10. Treatment of impetigo includes:

A. Giving IV antibiotics for 5 days to prevent sepsis
B. Removing crusts and applying alcohol to dry lesions
C. Removing crusts and applying antibiotic ointment
D. Giving oatmeal baths to treat itching and to dry lesions

11. The nits for pediculosis capitis (lice) are usually located:

A. On scalp and face
B. In axilla and groin
C. On hair shafts behind ears
D. In neck creases

12. Untreated cellulitis can lead to:

A. Otitis media
B. Osteomyelitis
C. Necrosis of skin
D. Neutropenia

13. A child with scabies will have:

    A. Infected lesions
    B. Intense pain
    C. Permanent scarring
    D. Intense pruritus

14. Parents of children taking broad-spectrum antibiotics should be cautioned to:

    A. Be alert for development of thrush
    B. Avoid giving child milk products
    C. Schedule follow-up visits to have blood levels drawn
    D. Have child eat diet high in iron

15. Second- and third-degree burns are more common in children because:

    A. Their skin has more water
    B. Their fight-or-flight response is immature
    C. Their skin is more sensitive
    D. They panic when burned

16. Anticipatory guidance about burns for parents of toddlers would include:

    A. Use cigarette lighters rather than matches for starting flames
    B. Keep pot handles turned in on stove
    C. Keep fireplace screen in place
    D. Keep child out of sunlight

17. A circumferential burn needs to be monitored carefully to avoid:

    A. Restriction of circulation
    B. Edema
    C. Major scarring
    D. Pressure points

18. Wound care usually includes the application of silver sulfadiazine cream because it is a:

    A. Corticosteroid cream that decreases edema
    B. Lubricant that keeps skin hydrated

    C. Silver compound that promotes new tissue growth
    D. Topical antibiotic that controls bacteria

19. After a child with major burns is discharged, continued care would include:

    A. Taking oral narcotics daily
    B. Low-calorie diet to prevent obesity
    C. Applying lotion daily to scars
    D. Wearing an elasticized garment

20. During a camping trip a Scout crawled out of his sleeping bag during the night and was found in the morning outside his tent. His lips were blue, his skin color was pale, he was confused, and he was breathing slowly. The best action to take while calling for help is:

    A. Wrap him in blanket
    B. Place him in sleeping bag with another camper
    C. Try to get him to drink warm fluids
    D. Briskly rub his arms and legs

21. A toddler is pulled from a river after falling through the ice. She was underwater for 30 minutes. CPR is begun at the site and continued:

    A. Until spontaneous respirations return
    B. Until she reaches hospital
    C. For 30 minutes
    D. Until body temperature returns to normal

22. If frostbite is suspected, initial care of the affected part includes:

    A. Rubbing area vigorously
    B. Exposure to warm air temperatures
    C. Immersion in warmed water
    D. Lowering affected part below level of heart

23. A child is bitten by a wild raccoon that escapes capture. It is essential that the following action be carried out:

    A. Wash wound carefully
    B. Administer antirabies serum

C. Warn child to avoid wild animals

D. Administer antibiotics

24. When a child is stung by a bee, he or she should be observed for:

A. Presence of fever

B. Joint pressure

C. Severe itching

D. Possible anaphylaxis

25. The appropriate treatment after a child sustains a possible contusion is to:

A. Observe for swelling

B. Immobilize injured area

C. Apply ice to area

D. Apply heat to area

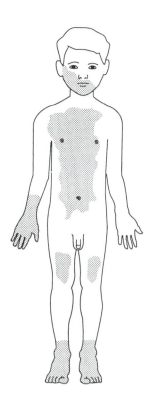

CASE STUDIES

1. Janice, 14 years old, has eczema. She is experiencing a flare-up with lesions on her face, neck, arms, and feet. Although it is summer, Janice is wearing makeup, wool pants, and a turtleneck sweater. Her skin appears dry. Outline an education plan for Janice to help control this irritation.

2. Matthew, 3 years old, was playing cowboy when he became curious about what his mother was cooking on the stove. He grabbed the handle of a deep-fat fryer, pulling it off the stove and pouring hot oil down his face, chest, and abdomen and into his boots. He was wearing a vest, jeans, and cowboy boots with no socks. Matthew's mother immediately poured cold water on his face and body but did not realize until later that the oil had also poured into Matthew's boots.
   A. Using the accompanying drawing of the burned areas, estimate the percentage of Matthew's body surface area (BSA) that has been burned.
   B. Outline a plan of care for Matthew.

Suggested Learning Activities

1. Visit a burn center that treats children.
   A. What are their standard protocols for burn care?
   B. Do family members participate in care?
   C. Is there a play therapist on the staff?
   D. What family supports are present?
   E. Are there active support groups for parents and children? Request to visit a group to observe the concerns that are expressed and the support that is given by the group.

2. Visit a local elementary school and meet with the school nurse. Some areas to investigate may include:
   A. Are children screened for head lice? How is the screening performed? What procedure is followed if lice are found? When can the child return to school?
   B. How are impetigo, athlete's foot, and ringworm handled in the schools? Are the children isolated?
   C. What action is taken if a child is bitten by another child or animal while at school?

ANSWERS WITH RATIONALES

Review of Concepts

COMPLETION

1. Secondary Skin Lesions

Lesion Name	Example
A. Crust	Impetigo
B. Scale	Dandruff
C. Lichenification	Eczema
D. Scar	Healed surgical incision
E. Keloid	Healed skin area after traumatic injury
F. Excoriation	Scratched insect bite
G. Fissure	Tinea pedis (athlete's foot)
H. Erosion	Ruptured chicken pox vesicle
I. Ulcer	Chancre

2. Tinea Infections

Type	Site	Clinical Manifestions
A. Tinea capitis	Scalp	Hair loss (one or several patches), broken hairs, thickened white scales, fine scaling
B. Tinea corporis	Trunk	One or several circular erythematous patches, may be scaly or erythematous throughout
C. Tinea cruris	Inner thighs, inguinal creases ("jock itch")	Scaly erythematous eruption, possibly elevated lesions, possible papules or vesicles
D. Tinea pedis	Feet and toes ("athlete's foot")	Vesicles or erosions on instep or between toes (fissures, red scaly)

MATCHING

1.

1. A, D
2. A, B, C
3. A
4. A, B, C
5. A, B, C

1. Allergic contact dermatitis is an inflammation of the skin that occurs in response to an allergen. Some common allergens are poison ivy, poison oak, rubber, shoe leather, and nickel. Symptoms can develop up to 18 hours after contact, peak between 48 and 72 hours after contact, and can last up to 3 weeks.

   Irritant contact dermatitis is an inflammation of the skin that occurs in response to an irritant. Common irritants include soaps, detergents, bleaches, lotions, urine, and stool. Symptoms develop within a few hours of contact, peak within 24 hours, and quickly resolve.

2. Diaper rash can be caused by urine, stool, diaper wipes, and detergents. To decrease the skin irritation, parents should be advised to:
   A. Change diapers often so there is less contact with stool and urine.
   B. Wash the perianal area with warm water and a mild soap with every diaper change.
   C. Expose the skin to air if possible (place the baby on an absorbent pad with diaper off—for males, drape a cloth over the penis). After air exposure apply A&D ointment, zinc oxide, Desitin, or Balmex to the skin to provide protection from the acidity of urine and stool.
   D. Avoid using rubber pants.
   E. Use only mild detergents and soaps and rinse cloth diapers a second time in the wash cycle.
   F. Avoid commercial baby wipes that contain alcohol, which can make the rash worse.
   G. Use superabsorbent disposable diapers that keep the skin drier.

3. Emphasize that anyone can get lice. Discuss the following interventions with the parents:
   A. Wash the child's hair with a pediculicide shampoo and a small amount of water. Rub the lather into the scalp for 4–5 minutes, and then rinse out thoroughly. Take care to avoid getting shampoo in the child's eyes. Next, remove the nits (eggs) with a fine-toothed comb soaked in vinegar. If nits still adhere to the hair, apply a vinegar compress for 15 minutes and then recomb. Repeat this procedure in 7 days.
   B. Nits that are shed hatch in 8–10 days; therefore, change the child's bedding and clothing daily, launder in hot water, and dry in a hot dryer for 20 minutes. Store other bedding and clothing in a tightly sealed bag for 10 days to 2 weeks, and then launder. Wash hairbrushes and combs with a pediculicide, soak in boiling water for 10–15 minutes, or discard. Vacuum furniture and treat with a hot iron when possible.
   C. All the child's contacts, including family members, should be examined and treated as necessary. Be certain that the school and day care facility are notified so that all children can be examined.

4. Burn severity is determined by depth of burn injury, percentage of body surface area (BSA) affected, and involvement of specific body parts (genitals, face, etc.).

5. Burn depth is described as:
   A. *Partial-thickness*—The injured tissue can regenerate and heal (first- and second-degree burns).
   B. *Full-thickness*—The injured tissue cannot regenerate (third-degree burns). This type of burn requires skin grafting.

6. A whirlpool bath is used before debridement to loosen eschar, to increase vasodilation and circulation, and to speed healing.

7. The four types of grafts are:
   A. *Autograft*—Healthy skin that is taken from the child's own body to cover the burned area. This type of graft is permanent.
   B. *Allograft*—A temporary graft that uses skin from a cadaver. (*Note:* There is a potential risk of HIV infection when using tissue from another person.)
   C. *Xenograft*—A temporary graft that uses skin from another species (e.g., pig skin).
   D. *Synthetic*—A temporary graft that uses artificial skin substances.

8. Play therapy for children:
   A. Provides an outlet for frustration, independence, and creativity.
   B. Promotes activities that challenge range of motion.

C. Normalizes daily routine.

D. Encourages the child who sees the progress that other children make day by day.

9. Repeated sunburns can lead to skin damage and cancer. Ways to prevent sunburn include:

A. Keep children out of direct sunlight as much as possible. Be aware that water, concrete, and sand reflect sunlight and increase exposure up to 90%.

B. Avoid exposure between 10 AM and 2 PM.

C. Use sunscreen of 15 SPF (sun protection factor) or greater on all exposed areas. Reapply every 2 hours as needed. Use a waterproof sunscreen when swimming.

D. Recognize that burns can still occur on cloudy days.

E. Minimize exposed areas when outdoors by using hats and long-sleeved shirts and leaving T-shirts on while swimming.

(*Note:* If a child is taking medications, check to see if hypersensitivity to sunlight is a side effect.)

Critical Thinking: Application/Analysis

MULTIPLE CHOICE

1. C. The newborn has thin skin with little subcutaneous fat, resulting in more rapid loss of heat, greater difficulty regulating body temperature, and more rapid chilling.

2. A. Cradle cap can usually be prevented with proper scalp hygiene. The hair should be washed daily with a gentle shampoo. Many parents do not wash the scalp because they fear putting pressure on or injuring the infant's "soft spot." Reassure parents that gentle cleansing will not harm the infant.

3. C. Topical corticosteroids are the treatment of choice for areas other than the scalp.

4. B. Children can develop a drug allergy to a new drug within 7 days. The most common reactions are rashes and hives. These should be reported, and the drug should be stopped immediately.

5. D. A family history of hay fever, asthma, or contact dermatitis frequently predisposes a child to eczema.

6. A. A mild soap will decrease irritation to the skin.

7. C. Touching and squeezing the lesions can introduce bacteria and injure the skin around the lesions.

8. A. Vitamin A preparations can make the skin sensitive to sunlight, resulting in sunburns with even minimal exposure.

9. D. Cystic acne is treated with oral antibiotics, vitamin A, and benzoyl peroxide. The goal of treatment is to prevent infection and scarring, and to minimize psychological distress.

10. C. The crusts must be removed to treat the infected lesions with antibiotic ointment. These lesions are caused by an infection with streptococci and/or staphylococci, which necessitates treatment with an antibiotic.

11. C. The eggs (nits) are laid on the hair shaft close to the scalp. Nits are found most often behind the ears and at the back of the head.

12. B. Cellulitis is an infection of the skin and subcutaneous fat that can lead to serious complications if untreated or if treatment is inadequate. Possible complications are osteomyelitis, arthritis, sepsis, and abscesses.

13. D. Intense pruritus is caused by sensitization to the ova and mite feces, which occurs approximately 1 month after infestation with scabies.

14. A. Broad-spectrum antibiotics can kill the normal flora in the body, permitting overgrowth of fungi such as *Candida albicans*.

15. C. Because children have thin sensitive skin, the time it takes to inflict a second- or third-degree burn is very short.

16. B. Many toddlers suffer scald burns from pulling hot liquids onto themselves, usually from a table or stove. Keep pot handles turned in so the child cannot pull them down.

17. A. Severe burns develop a layer of eschar (a tough leathery scab) over the burned area. Eschar that completely surrounds an arm or leg has no elasticity. If edema should occur, circulation could be cut off to the limb. An escharotomy (incision into the eschar) would then be necessary to restore peripheral circulation.

18. D. Because circulation is disrupted in the burned tissues, systemic antibiotics are not very useful in killing bacteria in wounds. Silver sulfadiazine (Silvadeen) cream is a topical antibiotic.

19. D. An elasticized (Jobst) garment is worn at all times to decrease the scarring.

20. B. Contact with the warm child will stop heat loss from the victim and begin to warm him by skin-to-skin contact.

21. D. This child has lost body heat (hypothermia) in the water. The diving reflex occurs when the face and nose are immersed in cold water, and the blood is shunted from the extremities to the vital organs, conserving oxygen. Resuscitation measures should continue until the body temperature reaches normal because the diving reflex may have preserved the vital organs.

22. C. Rewarming is done slowly to decrease the chance of cellular damage. Immerse the part for 10–15 minutes in water warmed to between 100° and 105°F (37.8° and 40.5°C).

23. B. Many wild animals are infected with rabies. Anyone who is bitten by an animal that cannot be observed or tested for rabies must receive rabies vaccination. Rabies is nearly 100% fatal to humans. (Refer to Chapter 10.)

24. D. A child previously sensitized can have an anaphylactic reaction to a bee sting. If sensitivity is known, the child should carry injectable epinephrine.

25. C. Contusions are soft tissue injuries that can result in swelling, pain, and infection. Applying ice soon after the injury can reduce inflammation and swelling.

CASE STUDIES

1. There is no cure for eczema; however, the condition can be controlled. Some measures to take are avoiding abrasive detergents, fabric softeners, cosmetics, perfumed lotions and soaps, and abrasive clothing such as wool. These can increase the skin irritation and lead to more intense itching (pruritus). Janice needs to avoid scratching the lesions because this can cause them to become infected and possibly result in permanent scarring. To lubricate her dry skin, lotion can be applied after bathing. An emollient (Eucerin) can be applied to noninflamed areas. To reduce inflammation, topical corticosteroids (hydrocortisone 1% or triamcinolone 0.1% ointments) can be applied one to three times daily for 4–5 days. To help with itching, the physician may order an antipruritic (Vistaril). Humidification in winter and air conditioning in the summer will also help.

   Janice is probably very upset about her appearance. Many of the lesions are visible on her face, neck, and arms, and she is trying to hide them under makeup and clothing. Explain that wearing cosmetics can make her eczema worse. She will need emotional support because she probably fears her peers' response to the lesions. Reassure Janice that the lesions are not contagious and will not result in scarring. Explain that she can reduce the flare-ups by following the recommendations outlined. The knowledge that she can control the eczema can help to increase her self-confidence.

2. A. Using the Lund and Browder chart for determining percentage of BSA in pediatric burn injuries, the following percentages of burns were estimated: face 3%, chest and abdomen 9%, right hand and forearm 2¾%, thighs 4%, ankles and feet 6%, for a total of 24¾% of BSA burned. This indicates that Matthew has suffered a ma-

jor (greater than 15%) burn. Other factors that increase the severity are the involvement of the face, the anterior chest, one hand, and both feet, because there is a potential for functional impairment in these areas. Matthew has third-degree burns on his feet and second-degree burns in other areas.

B. Because of the burns on Matthew's face, there is a potential for airway compromise. Initial care involves assessment of ABCs (airway, breathing, circulation). Fluid replacement is begun, usually with lactated Ringer's solution, to prevent hypovolemic shock. The plan of care for Matthew should include:

1. *Control pain*—Assess pain using the Faces scale (see Chapter 7). Cover burns. Use analgesics during dressing changes and to promote sleep. Elevate right hand and both feet on pillows to reduce swelling and pain. Provide diversional activities to lessen focus on pain. Change position often. Exercise feet and hand.

2. *Prevent infection*—Assess for fever. Use protective isolation when burns are open and sterile technique for dressing changes. Limit visitors and admit no one to visit who is ill. Debride necrotic tissue. Apply topical antibacterial agents. Cover burns with sterile dressings.

3. *Maintain fluid balance*—Monitor capillary refill time, intake and output, and daily weight. Administer fluids as ordered intravenously and orally. Monitor for hyponatremia and hyperkalemia.

4. *Decrease edema in burned extremities*—Elevate right hand and both feet on pillows. Check pedal and radial pulses every hour.

5. *Maintain airway patency*—Monitor respirations, breath sounds, and pulse oximetry. Elevate head of bed. Keep intubation tray at bedside.

6. *Maintain joint motion*—Perform range of motion exercises twice daily for right hand and both feet. Splint hand and feet if necessary.

7. *Maintain adequate nutrition*—Give nasogastric (NG) feedings if ordered. Weigh daily. Offer a variety of foods. Give a multivitamin supplement.

8. *Decrease child's anxiety*—Assign the same caregivers when possible. Encourage parents to bring familiar objects and pictures from home and to stay at the hospital and bedside.

9. *Decrease parent's anxiety*—Educate the parents about burn care and grafting. Refer the parents to social services or to a support group.

ALTERATIONS IN
PSYCHOSOCIAL FUNCTION

Chapter Overview

Chapter 22 focuses on alterations in psychosocial function in children. General psychotherapeutic management of children is discussed, including treatment modes, therapeutic strategies, and the nurse's role in both inpatient and community settings. Specific disorders presented include autistic disorder, attention deficit hyperactivity disorder (ADHD), mental retardation, eating and elimination disorders, substance abuse, depression and anxiety, childhood schizophrenia, conversion reaction, and child abuse. Each disorder is described, along with its medical and nursing management.

Learning Objectives

After studying this chapter, you should be able to:
- Describe the various treatment modes and therapeutic strategies used to treat children and adolescents with psychosocial disorders.
- Discuss the characteristic behaviors and the medical and nursing management of children who are autistic.
- Describe the characteristic behaviors of a child with ADHD.
- Discuss the care of mentally retarded children in the hospital and the community.
- Describe feeding disorder of infancy or early childhood and outline nursing management of children with this disorder.
- Discuss the care of children with encopresis.
- Differentiate between anorexia nervosa and bulimia nervosa.
- Discuss the medical and nursing management of adolescents with anorexia nervosa and bulimia nervosa.
- List commonly abused drugs and their effects.
- Describe various clinical manifestations of substance abuse.
- Describe characteristic findings of depression and anxiety in children and adolescents.
- Outline risk factors for suicide in children and adolescents.
- Discuss separation anxiety and school phobia and the nursing management of children with these disorders.
- Describe the clinical manifestations of childhood schizophrenia and conversion reaction.
- Recognize the types of child abuse.
- Discuss the nursing management of children who have been abused.
- Discuss the nurse's role in reporting child abuse.
- Describe Munchausen syndrome by proxy and outline the nursing management of children with this disorder.

Review of Concepts

COMPLETION

1. Commonly Abused Drugs and Their Effects

Drug	Effects of Intoxication
A. Alcohol	
B. Amphetamines	
C. Heroin	
D. LSD (lysergic acid diethylamide)	
E. Marijuana	

MATCHING

Match the items in list 1 with the appropriate word or phrase in list 2. (*Note:* Items may be used more than once.)

1. Eating Disorders

LIST 1
A. Anorexia nervosa
B. Bulimia nervosa
C. Compulsive overeating and obesity

LIST 2
1. ____ Bingeing and purging
2. ____ Excessive compulsive exercising
3. ____ Low self-esteem
4. ____ Erosion of tooth enamel
5. ____ Amenorrhea
6. ____ Distorted body image
7. ____ Esophagitis
8. ____ Electrolyte disturbances

2. Types of Child Abuse and Neglect

LIST 1
A. Physical abuse
B. Physical neglect
C. Emotional abuse
D. Emotional neglect
E. Sexual abuse
F. Munchausen by proxy

LIST 2
1. ____ Fondling genitals
2. ____ Lack of personal attention from parent
3. ____ Hitting child
4. ____ Lack of clean clothes
5. ____ Telling child "You're worthless"
6. ____ Feigned illness in healthy child
7. ____ Parental coldness toward child
8. ____ Oral-genital contact
9. ____ Tying child to furniture
10. ____ Inadequate winter clothes
11. ____ Harming child's pet

SHORT ESSAY

1. Identify five therapeutic strategies for working with children.

2. Describe the nursing measures needed to provide appropriate care to a mentally retarded child during hospitalization.

3. Describe the treatment to restore normal defecation in a child with encopresis.

4. Describe the binge-purge cycle that occurs in bulimia nervosa.

5. Describe the physical signs and symptoms that may lead a nurse to suspect substance abuse in an adolescent.

6. Describe the symptoms that may be noted in alcohol withdrawal.

7. Describe the clinical manifestations of major depression in children and adolescents.

8. List risk factors for suicide in children and adolescents.

9. Identify the characteristic behaviors of a child with schizophrenia.

10. Discuss the manifestations of emotional abuse seen in children.

Critical Thinking: Application/Analysis

MULTIPLE CHOICE

Select the best answer.

1. A type of therapy that is particularly effective with adolescents is:

   A. Play therapy
   B. Individual therapy
   C. Family therapy
   D. Group therapy

2. Play therapy is used to:

   A. Teach children how to play
   B. Help children to act out their feelings
   C. Help shy children to be creative
   D. Evaluate children's intelligence

3. A characteristic of autistic children is:

   A. Extreme aversion to touch
   B. Constant imitation of others
   C. Continual desire to be held
   D. Extreme interest in others

4. When a child with autism is admitted to the hospital, an appropriate nursing action would be to:

   A. Encourage other children to visit
   B. Isolate child from other children

   C. Decrease environmental stimuli
   D. Vary routines daily to maintain interest

5. When children who normally take Cylert for ADHD are admitted to the hospital, they should be:

   A. Given normal dose each day
   B. Allowed to stop medication in hospital
   C. Given increased dose in hospital
   D. Switched to different stimulant

6. A possible cause of feeding disorder of infancy is:

   A. Gastroesophaegeal reflux
   B. Cystic fibrosis
   C. Mental retardation
   D. Maternal neglect

7. Recurrent abdominal pain is the most commonly reported symptom of children who:

   A. Have irritable bowel syndrome
   B. Are afraid of unfamiliar places
   C. Are extremely shy
   D. Have been sexually abused

8. A characteristic often seen in families of girls with anorexia nervosa is parents who are:

   A. Overcontrolling
   B. Self-indulgent
   C. Abusive
   D. Loving and caring

9. Anorexia nervosa can be life threatening because it may result in:

   A. Respiratory compromise
   B. Dehydration
   C. Cardiac arrhythmias
   D. Immune system dysfunction

10. A serious complication of bulimia nervosa is:

    A. Cardiac arrhythmias
    B. Dehydration
    C. Dental caries
    D. Esophageal tears

11. A risk factor for depression and anxiety in children and adolescents is:

    A. Recent acute illness
    B. Family history of depression
    C. Above-average intelligence
    D. Attending a new school

12. A depressed child tells you he feels sad. How would you respond to him?

    A. "When do you get this sad feeling?"
    B. "Who makes you feel sad?"
    C. "Did your mother make you sad?"
    D. "You should be happy, not sad."

13. Many suicide attempts by children go unrecognized because adults:

    A. Expect children to engage in risky behaviors
    B. Don't believe children have reason to kill themselves
    C. Never ask child how injury happened
    D. Believe gesture will never be repeated

14. School phobia is often the result of a child's fear of:

    A. Failing in classroom
    B. Being embarrassed at school
    C. Leaving parent
    D. Riding school bus

15. Children are at higher risk for being physically abused if:

    A. They live in rural area
    B. They have several siblings
    C. Their parents were abused as children
    D. Their parents are divorced

16. An example of physical neglect is failure to:

    A. Send child to school
    B. Permit child to watch TV
    C. Attend to child for period of time
    D. Give prescribed medication

17. Children who withdraw accusations of abuse have usually been:

    A. Coerced into doing so
    B. Lying all along
    C. Mistakenly identified as victims of abuse
    D. Threatened into making initial accusation

18. In Munchausen syndrome, signs and symptoms of a health condition in a child are:

    A. Not recognized
    B. Fabricated
    C. Ignored
    D. Exaggerated

CASE STUDIES

1. Joshua, 8 years old, is admitted to the hospital with a fractured left tibia and femur. His injuries were incurred when he ran in front of a car while playing baseball. He has been placed in 90–90 skeletal traction and is very restless. His history reveals that he has ADHD and is receiving methylphenidate (Ritalin). What issues need to be addressed in the hospital care of Joshua?

2. Tom, 2½ years old, is admitted to the hospital with severe burns on the palm of his right hand. Tom's parents state that he climbed up on a stool when his mother was cooking supper and accidentally placed his hand in the gas flame while reaching for something. After admission, a nurse asks Tom how he hurt his hand, and he says, "Daddy put it in the fire. I peed my pants again and he got mad."

   The parents are interviewed again, and Tom's father admits that he burned his son's hand. The second interview reveals that the mother is usually at home with Tom and his two siblings. However, the father has recently lost his job and is now often at home during the day. Tension is very high in the household. The father is extremely domineering and does not allow his wife out of the house alone. He also admits to having had "a few drinks" the day of the abuse.

A. What is the nurse's responsibility once Tom makes his disclosure?

B. What factors in the family history and events surrounding the abuse are considered risk factors for abuse?

C. What nursing care is needed for Tom and his family?

Suggested Learning Activities

1. Obtain permission and attend a meeting of a self-help group that has adolescent members (e.g., Ala-Teen, Nar Anon). Observe the group process. How does the group function? What direction is given? What supports are evident? Interview several members of the group to determine what benefits they get from attending.

2. Interview a psychologist, psychiatrist, or pediatrician who evaluates children for ADHD. Areas to explore include:

A. How are these children referred for testing?

B. What tests are given?

C. If the diagnosis is confirmed, what is the treatment of choice?

D. What is the average age of patients?

E. Are there adolescent or adult patients?

ANSWERS WITH RATIONALES

Review of Concepts

COMPLETION

1. Commonly Abused Drugs and Their Effects

Drug	Effects of Intoxication
A. Alcohol	Decreased muscle tone and coordination; impaired speech, memory, and judgment; confusion; emotional lability
B. Amphetamines	Dilated pupils; increased pulse and blood pressure; flushing; nausea; euphoria; increased alertness; agitation, or irritability; hallucinations; insomnia
C. Heroin	Analgesia; depressed respirations and muscle tone; nausea; constricted pupils; changes in mood; drowsiness; impaired attention or memory; sense of tranquility
D. LSD (lysergic acid diethylamide)	Lack of coordination; dilated pupils; hypertension; elevated temperature; visual illusions and hallucinations; altered perceptions of time and space; emotional lability; psychosis
E. Marijuana	Tachycardia; reddened conjunctiva; dry mouth; increased appetite; initial anxiety followed by euphoria; giddiness; impaired attention, judgment, and memory

MATCHING

1.
1. B	2. A	3. A, B, C
4. B	5. A	6. A, B, C
7. B	8. A, B	

2.
1. E	2. D	3. A
4. B	5. C	6. F
7. D	8. E	9. A
10. B	11. C	

SHORT ESSAY

1. Five therapeutic strategies for working with children are play therapy, art therapy, behavior therapy, visualization and guided imagery, and hypnosis.

2. When a mentally retarded child is admitted to the hospital, the nurse should interview the parents to identify the child's abilities and special needs and to determine how the family manages the child's care at home. The child's current abilities and skills, such as toileting and feeding, should be assessed and efforts to maintain these skills supported during hospitalization. The parents should be involved in the child's care as much as they desire. Interaction with the child should occur at his or her cognitive level. Socialization should be promoted by encouraging interaction between the child and other children on the unit.

3. Children with encopresis retain stool in the bowel, leading to constipation or diarrhea. When the bowel is impacted with stool, the liquid stool entering the large intestine continues through the intestine and is excreted as semiliquid stool. This often misleads parents into thinking the child is having diarrhea. Treatment involves emptying the bowel of impacted stool with lubricants and laxatives and increasing fiber and fluids in the diet. Once the bowel is empty,

appropriate toileting habits are encouraged by means of behavior modification. It will take several months for the muscle tone in the large intestine to return to normal. If the encopresis is psychological in origin, psychotherapy for the child and family is begun.

4. A bulimic adolescent often binges after a stressful event. At first the episodes of binge eating are pleasurable. Immediately after the binge episode, however, feelings of guilt, shame, anger, depression, fear of loss of control, and fear of weight gain arise. As these feelings intensify, the bulimic adolescent becomes increasingly anxious. This usually initiates the purge behaviors, which relieve the feelings of depression and guilt, but only temporarily.

5. Signs and symptoms of substance abuse include bloodshot eyes, dilated pupils, slurred speech, and weight loss. The substance abuser may appear sleepy or restless or may show signs of clumsiness or inconsistent behavior.

6. Symptoms of alcohol withdrawal include anxiety, headache, tremors, nausea and vomiting, malaise or weakness, tachycardia, hypertension, insomnia, depressed mood or irritability, and hallucinations.

7. Characteristic findings of major depression are declining school performance, withdrawal from social activities, sleep disturbance, appetite disturbance, multiple somatic complaints (e.g., headaches and stomachaches), and various conduct and behavioral problems.

8. Risk factors for childhood suicide are:
   A. School problems
   B. Pregnancy
   C. Drug use or abuse
   D. Problems with a romantic relationship
   E. Feelings of anxiety
   F. History of chronic family problems
   G. Chronic illness
   H. Physical, emotional, or sexual abuse
   I. History of suicide in a family member
   J. History of depression
   K. Chronic low self-esteem

9. Characteristic behaviors in childhood schizophrenia include social withdrawal, impaired social relationships, flat affect, regression, loose associations, delusions, and hallucinations.

10. Manifestations of emotional abuse, verbal abuse, and emotional neglect include fear, poor physical growth, and failure to meet appropriate developmental milestones. The child may also difficulty relating to adults, impaired communication skills, and developmental delays.

Critical Thinking: Application/Analysis

MULTIPLE CHOICE

1. D. Group therapy is effective with adolescents because of the importance of the peer group at this age.

2. B. Children who are experiencing anxiety and stress can act out their feelings of anger, hostility, sadness, and fear through play therapy. The therapist can also use play therapy to assist the child to understand his or her responses in a supportive environment.

3. A. Autistic children often respond abnormally to sensory stimuli such as touch, loud noises, and bright lights.

4. C. Autistic children respond to the environment differently from other individuals. Sounds that are not distressing to the average person may be interpreted by autistic children as louder, more frightening, or overwhelming. Encourage parents to bring favorite objects from home and try to keep these objects in the same places, because the child does not cope well with changes in the environment.

5. A. Cylert is a stimulant used in treatment of ADHD that can take 2–4 weeks to achieve a desired response. If the medication is discontinued in the hospital, the child is at risk of behavioral problems for several weeks after the drug is restarted.

6. D. Feeding disorder of infancy includes the pathologic refusal of food, sleep and feeding disorders, and social and emotional factors that interfere with adequate nutrition. It may reflect a lack of adequate maternal care and warmth.

7. D. The abdominal pain is probably due in part to the anxiety response but is often the symptom reported by children who have been sexually abused or traumatized in some way and is often a complaint of anxious or depressed children.

8. A. Many girls with anorexia nervosa come from dysfunctional families in which parents are over-controlling and perfectionistic.

9. C. Severe malnutrition leads to electrolyte imbalances and hyperkalemia, which can cause fatal cardiac arrhythmias.

10. D. Repeated bingeing and purging can cause esophageal tears.

11. B. A family history of depression, suicide, substance abuse, alcoholism, or other psychopathology is a risk factor for depression and anxiety in children and adolescents.

12. A. It is necessary to be accepting and nonjudgmental about any feelings expressed by a depressed child. Assist the child to identify any precipitating event when feelings of sadness arise.

13. B. Suicide gestures by children and adolescents are often labeled as "accidents." Adults may have difficulty believing that young children would have any reason to want to end their lives.

14. C. The child's fear of going to school is often a manifestation of his or her fear of leaving the parent or primary caregiver (usually the mother).

15. C. Children are at risk for physical abuse if their parents were abused as children.

16. D. Neglect involves an act of omission. Appropriate medical care is a basic need. Thus, deliberate withholding of prescription medication constitutes physical neglect.

17. A. Children usually do not make false allegations. When they rescind an accusation, they have usually been threatened or coerced into doing so.

18. B. In Munchausen syndrome the abuser (most often the mother) creates fictitious signs in her child to gain access to the medical system in order to meet her own needs. The child often appears anxious, fearful, and negative, whereas the caretaker, who thrives in the health care environment, is cooperative, competent, and loving. The child undergoes many tests, the results of which are all negative. After repeated admissions, the caretaker comes under suspicion because the symptoms appear only in her presence.

CASE STUDIES

1. Children with ADHD exhibit behaviors of inattention, impulsiveness, and hyperactivity. These children are usually admitted to the hospital for reasons other than ADHD (e.g., injuries, illness); however, the ADHD has a significant impact on their care and treatment.

   Joshua's fracture is the result of his impulsiveness. He is restless in bed, and it may be difficult to determine whether the cause is pain or short attention span. Safety concerns include (1) whether Joshua will be able to stay still in bed and keep his traction in appropriate alignment, and (2) whether he will be able to avoid playing with the traction pin and causing an infection. (ADHD children have been known to fall out of bed while in traction when reaching for objects and have caused osteomyelitis in the pin site by contaminating the wounds or sliding the pin back and forth.) If not contraindicated, Joshua should receive his normal dosage of Ritalin during his hospital stay. This will help to control his impulsiveness and hyperactivity while improving his attention span. Be alert for side effects of anorexia, insomnia, and tachycardia. Work with both Joshua and his parents to set up a daily schedule and routine. Children with ADHD function better in a structured environment. Determine what disciplinary techniques are most effective at home and use them in the hospital if appropriate.

Praise Joshua's abilities and accomplishments. Children with ADHD often have poor self-esteem because of their impulsiveness and the problems it creates. Setting up a reward system using stickers or stars for positive behaviors or completed tasks is effective with many ADHD children. For teaching to be effective, schedule sessions after Joshua's Ritalin dose. Also, give only one instruction at a time.

2. A. Nurses are mandated by law to report to child protective services any suspected child abuse that is discovered in their work. (Nurses or other mandated reporters who do not report suspected abuse can be held responsible for their actions.) The nurse needs to record, in quotes, exactly what Tom and his parents say. Photographs should be taken of the injury and referral made to a specialist in child abuse.

B. Factors in this history that are considered risk factors for abuse are Tom's age, his father's drinking and loss of job, and his mother's social isolation and powerless position. Tom's father also has inappropriate expectations regarding his ability to be potty trained at age 2½.

C. Nursing care for Tom includes reassuring him that he did nothing wrong and is not to blame for his burn. To prevent further abuse, Tom should be placed in protective custody by social services while his injury is cared for in the hospital.

Tom's parents may stay away from the hospital because of fear and guilt. They need to be regularly updated on their child's progress, because they are still the child's primary caregivers. If they do visit, the medical and nursing staff need to be nonjudgmental and supportive. The parents should be encouraged to care for Tom while visiting and their interactions with their child observed and documented by staff.

A thorough evaluation of the home and family should be performed by an appropriate social services agency to determine whether returning to the home at discharge is appropriate. Tom could be returned home with supervised care or placed in foster care while decisions are being made about the family. Tom's parents may need referral to parenting classes, family therapy, or support groups.